Yoga Benefits Are in Breathing Less

Artour Rakhimov (PhD)

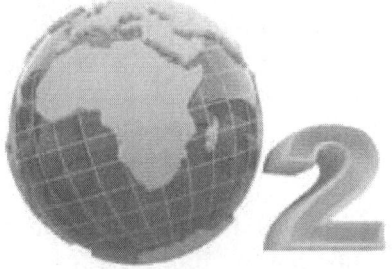

"All chronic pain, suffering and diseases are caused from a lack of oxygen at the cell level."

Guyton AC, The Textbook of Medical Physiology*, Fifth Edition.

* *World's most widely used medical textbook of any kind*

* *World's best-selling physiology book*

Copyright

Content copyright © Dr. Artour Rakhimov. All rights reserved - 2012.

This book is copyrighted. It is prohibited to copy, lend, adapt, electronically transmit, or transmit by any other means or methods without prior written approval from the author. However, the book may be borrowed by family members.

Disclaimer

The content provided herein is for information purposes only and not intended to diagnose, treat, cure or prevent cystic fibrosis or any other chronic disease. Always consult your doctor or health care provider before making any medical decisions). The information herein is the sole opinion of Dr. Artour Rakhimov and does not constitute medical advice. These statements have not been evaluated by Ontario Ministry of Health. Although every effort has been made to ensure the accuracy of the information herein, Dr. Artour Rakhimov accepts no responsibility or liability and makes no claims, promises, or guarantees about the accuracy, completeness, or adequacy of the information provided herein and expressly disclaims any liability for errors and omissions herein.

Content of the book

Introduction 1
   Who has special restrictions, limits,
   and temporary contraindications 3
1. Yoga and breathing 5
   1.1 The role of breathing in modern yoga 5
   1.2 Contemporary yoga leaders about breathing 6
   1.3 Traditional yoga about breathing 8
2. Physiology and medicine about normal breathing 11
   2.1 Physiological norms for breathing at rest 11
   2.2 Healthy people breathe very little 14
   2.3 Other parameters of normal breathing 17
3. You are likely a ... heavy breather 19
   3.1 Breathing in people with heart disease 19
   3.2 "Asthmatic" means a deep breather 22
   3.3 Deep breathing in people with diabetes 24
   3.4 People with other chronic diseases
   are also heavy breathers 26
   3.5 Over 90% of modern people,
   you probably included, breathe too much air 30
4. Effects of deep breathing (hyperventilation) 37
   4.1 Hypocapnia
   (or CO_2 deficiency in the blood and cells) 37
   4.2 Vasoconstriction 38
   4.3 Suppressed Bohr effect 43
   4.4 Less oxygen for cells 47
   4.5 CO_2 is crucial for mental health 50
   4.6 Other hypocapnia- and hypoxia-related effects 56
5. How to measure breathing and body oxygenation 59
   5.1 Could we measure total body O_2 using devices? 59
   5.2 Dr. Buteyko about yoga 62
   5.3 How to measure body O_2 (details) 64
   5.4 MCP (morning CP):
   your main health parameter 70
   5.4 Buteyko Table of Health Zones 71

6. Yoga benefits in relation to chronic diseases 79
   6.1 Respiratory diseases 79
   6.2 Cardiovascular diseases 81
   6.3 Hormonal conditions 83
   6.4 Gastrointestinal problems 84
   6.5 Diseases of kidneys and urinary tract 86
   6.6 Diseases of the musculoskeletal system 87
   6.7 Skin diseases 88
   6.8 Allergies and Immunodeficiency 89
7. Other yoga benefits due normalization of breathing 91
   7.1 Physiological and neurological changes 91
   7.2 General psychological and social changes 92
   7.3 Biochemical effects 93
   7.4 Technical skills 93
   7.5 Changes in physical and general sport skills 93
   7.6 Lifestyle changes as yoga benefits 94
8. Key practical steps in breathing retraining
to get yoga benefits 97
   Level 1. No exacerbations of chronic diseases 97
   Level 2. Stable health 97
   Level 3. Normal health 102
Conclusions 103

Introduction

Do you want to get am astonishing boost in your health and main yoga benefits using your usual yoga practice but combined together with one simple tip described in this book? This tip relates to the most important health factor: O2 content in the human body. Furthermore, this book will show you a simple DIY test that is very useful to use in order to monitor your progress in yoga and experience real yoga benefits. If you achieve a certain amount of oxygen in tissues of your vital organs, you will be free from about 200 chronic diseases that include heart disease, diabetes, cancer, asthma, bronchitis and many more. This book provides you with the most important parameters (including exact numbers) in your yoga practice: the direction where to go and the criteria that you need to achieve in order to, first, reduce and eliminate symptoms of common diseases, and, eventually, achieve real yoga health and practically experience yoga benefits (for more information, visit http://www.normalbreathing.com/yoga-benefits.php).

Yoga has always been about health especially physical health. For centuries, it was one of the most powerful techniques for physical rejuvenation. Probably, it was the most powerful technique for health restoration. Not anymore. You can practice yoga for months and years (the way it is now taught by leading yoga gurus), and your health may not improve or even can get worse. Why does modern yoga provides very limited benefits? Why was it successful in the past?

To put it simply, modern yoga leaders and yoga teachers do not know how to breathe! You can read tens of yoga books, and you will unlikely not find a single book on yoga that provides you exact numbers for ideal breathing even at rest of during sleep for maximum brain and body oxygenation. Furthermore, there is no goal in modern yoga. It is a purposeless eternal activity related to postures and exercise with some variations depending on yoga schools and their specific teachings. As about breathing, they say "breathe more", "breathe deeply", and many yoga gurus and teachers, can even add "expel toxic CO2". These are all inventions and fantasies of modern yoga teachers and mass media.

Traditional yoga never had such ideas. Their teaching was based on breathing slower and less. Furthermore, old yoga had a clear goal in mind, and this goal can found in many yoga books written centuries or many decades ago. There is factor that clearly separates sick and healthy people. Old yoga, without any scientific devices and measurement, grasped the essence of health. And yoga teachers in the past taught their pupils about this essence of yoga. But these days, using medical research, we can prove that old yoga was right.

Hundreds of medical studies have proved that chronic diseases are based on low levels on oxygen in body cells. What about breathing patterns in sick and healthy people? All available research, I am talking about hundreds of studies, has shown that sick people (heart disease, diabetes, cancer, asthma, bronchitis, COPD, and many other conditions) breathe about 2-3 times more air than the medical norm. They breathe deeply and expel "toxic CO2" exactly the way modern yoga gurus teach.

Even modern so called "normal subjects" breathe about 2 times more than the norm and much more than we used to breathe some during the first decades of the 20th century. When we breathe more air than the medical norm (it is called hyperventilation), we get less oxygen into our body cells. This is the law of physiology. Therefore, traditional yoga, and this book provides exact quotes from the most known ancient Sanskrit manuscripts, was absolutely right.

Virtually all traditional yoga practices are about better or slower breathing 24/7. Restoration of correct breathing defeats nearly all chronic diseases and leads to stunning level of health, no pain, no suffering, clarity of mind, joy of exercise, super short and very refreshing sleep (naturally down to a few hours only), and many other effects that comes with high body O2 content.

Note that this book does not provide all details that a yoga student requires to achieve good health. The book discusses the direction and expected results, as it was explained by Dr. Konstantin Buteyko.

Who has special restrictions, limits, and temporary contraindications

Breathing retraining and yoga breathing exercises (for more information, visit http://www.normalbreathing.com/yoga-breathing.php) produce a mild stress for the human body so that it needs to adapt to new conditions and function better in future. Such adaptive effects also take place during, for example, physical exercise. It would be silly for an unfit person to try to run a marathon without weeks or months of preparation.

If the demands due to yoga breathing exercises or other breathing exercises are too high, there is no adaptive response, and, as a result, the exercises can even produce a negative effect. Hence, breathing exercises should also be adjusted to the current adaptive abilities of the human organism. A more gradual approach in relation to hypoxic and hypercapnic demands of breathing exercises (quick changes in air composition) is necessary for many patients with:

- **Heart disease** (aortic aneurysms; angina pectoris; arrhythmia; atherosclerosis (plaque buildup); cardiomyopathy; ciliary arrhythmia (cardiac fibrillation); chest pain (angina pectoris); high cholesterol; chronic ischemia; congenital heart disease; congestive heart failure; coronary artery disease; endocarditis; extrasystole; heart murmurs; hypertension; hypertrophic cardiomyopathy; tachnycardia; pericarditis; post myocardial infarction; stroke)

- **Migraine headaches and panic attacks.** Those people, who recently had serious problems with their lungs or suffer from severe and moderate forms of lung damage, should avoid too fast and too large stretching (expansion or dilation) and shrinking (constriction) of their lungs. Hence, their inhalations and exhalations should be limited (not maximum) in their amplitude and velocity. This relates to people with:

- **Respiratory disorders involving the lungs** (asthma, bronchitis, COPD, emphysema, cystic fibrosis, pneumonia, tuberculosis; pulmonary edema; etc.)

Other specific situations include:
- **Presence of transplanted organs**
- **Pregnancy**
- **Brain traumas**
- **Acute bleeding injuries**
- **Blood clots**
- **Acute stages (exacerbations) of life-threatening conditions (infarct, stroke, cardiac ischemia, etc.)**
- **Insulin-dependent diabetes (type 2 diabetes)**
- **Loss of CO2 sensitivity.**

If you suffer from any of these conditions, you should follow special suggestions due to restrictions, limits, and temporary contraindications. These conditions do not prevent you from enjoying excellent health, but they impose some restrictions on your yoga practice.

Warning. *It is your responsibility, in cases of doubts to consult your family physician or GP about breathing retraining and use of yoga breathing exercises, as well as other breathing exercises, for your specific health problems. In addition, you need to consult your health care provider about your medication and any changes in dosages of medication.*

1. Yoga and breathing

1.1 The role of breathing in modern yoga

There are hundreds of yoga styles or different versions of yoga that exist worldwide. Many of these schools include or even emphasize that breathing is their important part.

Hatha Yoga is the most popular type of yoga and is the origin for many other yoga types and forms including Ashtanga Yoga and Power Yoga considered below. Hatha Yoga includes Pranayama and some other breathing exercises. The instructions and final goals for these exercises are different depending on location and teacher's understanding of yoga. However, the most common views of Hatha Yoga teachers are provided in the following part of this book together with views of other yoga teachers.

Another example of yoga is **Ashtanga Yoga** that suggests relaxed diaphragmatic breathing that is accompanied by sounds from the practitioner's throat. This breathing pattern is aligned with physical movements. This steady cycle of inhales and exhales provides the yoga student with a calming mental focal point.

BTS Iyengar invented his own movement or yoga style that is called **Iyengar Yoga**. It is also based on traditional Hatha Yoga and involves yoga asanas and breathing exercises.

Kriya Yoga is sometimes considered as a direct form of Yoga Therapy. The intention is to purify the body, but there is again no criterion for purification. There are many other forms of yoga that had they origins in Kriya Yoga.

Kundalini Yoga places focus of instruction on student's awareness of the energy centers throughout the body. It is based on a combination of yoga postures, Pranayama, and mantras. The intention is to transform the mind and emotions with some emphasis on yoga breath control. But this technique, as it is taught these days, also does not provide the student with clear goals and criteria of success.

Power Yoga is often known as the Westernized version of the Indian Ashtanga Yoga. It is popular in the Western world. Power Yoga is a physically challenging practice that involves yoga poses and breathing exercises with an intention to cleanse the body of toxins and negative (or destructive) emotions.

Hot Yoga or **Bikram Yoga** (for more information visit http://www.normalbreathing.com/yoga-breathing.php) includes 26 postures and two breathing exercises that are practiced in a hot room. A specific feature of Bikram Yoga is its surrounding temperature (about 40°C or over 105°F) and humidity (~40%) trying to mimic conditions in India.

Since oxygen to body cells is provided due to breathing, let us consider views of modern yoga leaders (for more information visit http://www.normalbreathing.com/yoga2.php) related to breathing .

1.2 Contemporary yoga leaders about breathing

First, we can look review written ideas and statements related to breathing that can be found in books written by modern yoga leaders in their books and internet sites devoted to yoga. What do they say about breathing.

There is literally nothing about breathing at all in one of the main Iyengar's book "*Yoga: The Path to Holistic Health*". There is an impression that he either does not how to breathe, or does not know how to explain this part of yoga practice.

The leaders of Hot Yoga movement Bikram Choudhury, in his main book "*Bikram Yoga*", devoted several pages to breathing. On page 99, in this book, there is a chapter called "Standing Deep Breathing" with a subtitle "First Breathing Exercises". The next four pages of the book are devoted to description of this breathing exercise. It is suggested to take the maximum (or "deeper and fuller") inhalation for six counts and then exhale for the same duration of time. This cycle is to be repeated 10 times. As about the progress, at the beginning, as Bikram Choudhury writes, a novice cannot get full inhalations and exhalations because the lungs are "tight and small". But after training, it becomes easier to do the same exercise since the hot yoga student is able to use their lungs more fully and pump more air using the same counting: 6 for inhalations and 6 for exhalations. The main purpose of this exercise, according to Bikram, is to use up to 100% of the lungs so that prevent respiratory problems, such as bronchitis, asthma, and emphysema.

This Section of Bikram's book also suggests that this is Pranayama breathing (visit http://www.normalbreathing.com/d/pranayama-benefits.php for more about pranayama benefits). The exercise may cause unusual symptoms, as he writes. Feeling of dizziness is common, but it should disappear. As Bikram explains, this sensation of dizziness is due to too much oxygen in the system. He also notes that it is important to keep one eye's open to prevent loss of balance and falling over during this breathing exercise.

There is an explanation of another exercise on page 205 that is called "Blowing in Firm Pose (Kapalbhati in Vajrasana)". During this exercise you the student is supposed to expel every ounce of carbon dioxide and replace it with oxygen. This is how one of the modern yoga leaders understands yoga breathing, Pranayama, and expected effects of breathing exercises. Later in this book, we are going to explore the expected effects of low CO2 (when one blows out carbon dioxide due to heavy breathing). We are also going to prove that all these negative symptoms (dizziness and a chance of fainting) are due to reduced levels of oxygen in the brain caused by hyperventilation.

Other yoga teachers that represent other forms and types of yoga generally have the same or similar ideas. During last several years, I spoke with various yoga teachers. Such conversations often could take place before or after my introductory lectures about breathing or in some other situations. Majority of yoga teachers, as soon as they start thinking about breathing, for some strange reasons, focus on breathing exercises and start to claim that breathing should be diaphragmatic and deep. Ask your yoga teachers about breathing. My strong impression, after reading dozens of modern yoga books and speaking with many yoga teachers is that nearly the whole community of yoga teachers lives with some weird obsession that "breathing" means "breathing exercises". Somehow, they assume that oxygen for body cells is required only during some 20, 40 or 60 minutes of yoga breathing exercises.

My views are that we require oxygen 24/7 or day and night. Therefore, we require to have correct breathing every minute of each day. Furthermore, when severely sick and terminally ill people die due to complications of diseases and acute exacerbations, their breathing becomes deeper and faster, while body brain and heart oxygenation becomes critically low. This effect, according to numerous medical studies, takes place during early morning hours (from about 4 until 7 am), and this is exactly the time that has highest mortality rates due to heart attacks, strokes, seizures, exacerbations of asthma, and many other complications.

Conclusions. There are following serious problems with such teaching of modern yoga leaders and teachers. First of all, yoga teachers assume that "breathing" means "breathing exercises", while, in reality, breathing is a continuous process to deliver oxygen all the time. Second, yoga teachers do not provide any information about ideal automatic (or unconscious) breathing that should be the goal of each and every yoga student.

References

Choudhury, Bikram, *Bikram Yoga*, HarperCollins Publishers, ISBN-10: 0-060-56808-5, 2007.

Iyengar, BKS, *Yoga: The Path to Holistic Health*, A Dorling Kindersley Book, ISBN 0-7894-7165-5, 2001

1.3 Traditional yoga about breathing

You probably also have heard that they say, "Take deep breath", ""Breathe deeper", and "Breathe more air" and can add, "You will get more oxygen in the cells". Do ancient hatha yoga manuscripts have the same ideas? Some of these books have been written up to 5 and more centuries ago. The main yoga books say that the goal of yoga breathing exercises is to "restrain", "hold", "suspend", and "calm" the breath days and nights. Here are quotes from 3 most important and most know yoga manuscripts: Hatha Yoga Pradipika, the Gheranda Samhita and the Shiva Samhita.

Hatha Yoga Pradipika (15 century)

"3. So long as the (breathing) air stays in the body, it is called life. Death consists in passing out of the (breathing) air. It is, therefore, necessary to restrain the breath."

"17. Hiccough, asthma, cough, pain in the head, the ears, and the eyes; these and other various kinds of diseases are generated by the disturbance of the breath."

The Shiva Samhita (17-18 century)

(5) The Pranayama

"22. Then let the wise practitioner close with his right thumb the pingala (right nostril), inspire air through the ida (the left nostril); and keep the air confined – suspend his breathing – as long as he can; and afterwards let him breathe out slowly, and not forcibly, through the right nostril. 23. Again, let him draw breath through the right nostril, and stop breathing as long as his strength permits; then let him expel the air through the left nostril, not forcibly, but slowly and gently."

"39. When the Yogi can, of his will, regulate the air and stop the breath (whenever and how long) he likes, then certainly he gets success in kumbhaka, and from the success in kumbhaka only, what things cannot the Yogi commend here?"

"43. ... from the perfection of pranayama, follows decrease of sleep, excrements and urine."

Increase of Duration

"53. Then gradually he should make himself able to practice for three gharis (one hour and a half at a time, he should be able to restrain breath for that period). Through this, the Yogi undoubtedly obtains all the longed for powers."

"57. When he gets the power of holding breath (i.e., to be in a trance) for three hours, then certainly the wonderful state of pratyahar is reached without fail."

The Gheranda Samhita (15-17 century)

"7. Wherever the yogi may be, he should always, in everything he does, be sure to keep the tongue upwards and constantly hold the breath. This is Nabhomudra, the destroyer of diseases for yogis."

The Yoga Sutra of Patanjali (4th-2nd century BC)

"Pranayama [the main breathing exercise in yoga] is the cessation of inspiratory and expiratory movements."

As it is easy to notice that classical yoga books say that we need to breathe less and hold our breath for better health. These traditional yoga ideas are exactly opposite to what modern yoga leaders and teachers promote. In classical yoga texts, there are no referrals to breathing more or expelling any toxins from the lungs. Who is right? It cannot be so that we experience the same effects in these 2 conditions:

1. when we breathe more air and expel "toxic" CO2 (as modern yoga teachers advise)
2. we hold the breath and restrain our breathing all the time (as traditional yoga taught).

How can we solve this argument? Obviously, if there is certain usual or normal breathing pattern in a healthy person, then breathing more than in normal conditions or less than in normal conditions should produce some effects on oxygen transport. What are the effects?

When we breathe more air and increase ventilation of the lungs at rest, we should accumulate more CO2 (carbon dioxide) in the airways, blood and other body cells. When we breathe less air, CO2 rises. These physiological effects have been studied in hundreds of studies. What are the effects of changes in CO2 levels on oxygen delivery to cells of the body? If we find the answers to these questions, then we can decide who provides correct ideas (traditional yoga or modern yoga leaders and teachers). In addition, this knowledge can be used in practice in order to improve body oxygenation and overall health.

2. Physiology and medicine about normal breathing

Let us start with medical norms for breathing at rest, as well as typical respiratory parameters in healthy, ordinary and sick people.

2.1 Physiological norms for breathing at rest

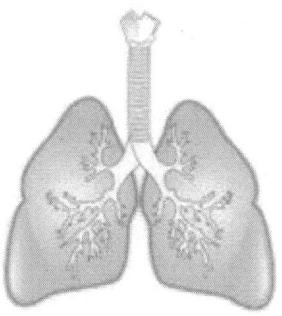

Normal breathing is strictly nasal (for inhalations and exhalations), predominantly diaphragmatic (i.e., up to 80-90% abdominal), very slow in frequency (about 12 breaths per minute) and imperceptible (no feelings or sensation about one's own breathing at rest since it is very small or unnoticeable). **The physiological norm for minute ventilation at rest is 6 liters of air for one minute for a 70 kg man**, as numerous physiological textbooks indicate (e.g., Guyton, 1984; Ganong, 1995; and Straub, 1998). These medical textbooks also provide the following parameters for normal breathing:
- normal breathing frequency is about 12 breaths per minute
- normal tidal volume (air volume breathed in during a single breath) is 500 ml
- normal inspiration is about 2 seconds
- normal exhalation is about 3 seconds.

Yoga Benefits are in Breathing Less

To be more accurate, the normal inhalation is little bit shorter or about 1.5 seconds, while the exhalation is longer or nearly 3.5 seconds. The following graph below represents the normal breathing (for more information, visit http://www.normalbreathing.com) pattern at rest. The graph shows changes in air volume in the lungs as a function of time at rest in an adult.

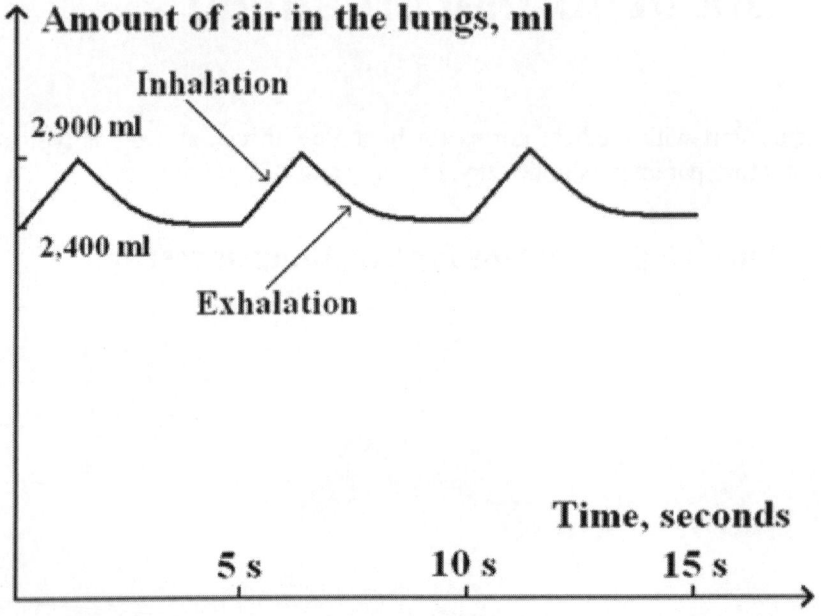

As it is noted above, if a person with normal breathing is asked about what they feel or their breathing sensations, they will testify that they do not feel their breathing at all (unless their practice yoga breathing or some other breathing exercises). Why could it be so? The normal tidal volume is only 500 ml or about 0.6 g (0.02 ounce) of air, which is inhaled during one inspiration. This is indeed a very small amount.

References (Medical and physiological textbooks)

Ganong WF, *Review of medical physiology*, 15-th ed., 1995, Prentice Hall Int., London.

Guyton AC, *Physiology of the human body*, 6-th ed., 1984, Suanders College Publ., Philadelphia.

Straub NC, *Section V, The Respiratory System, in Physiology*, eds. RM Berne & MN Levy, 4-th edition, Mosby, St. Louis, 1998.

Summary of values useful in pulmonary physiology: man. Section: Respiration and Circulation, ed. by P.L. Altman & D.S. Dittmer, 1971, Bethesda, Maryland (Federation of American Societies for Experimental Biology).

2.2 Healthy people breathe very little

We see that, according to these 14 recent medical studies, healthy people still breathe very small amount of air at rest.

Table. Minute ventilation at rest in healthy subjects

Condition	Minute ventilation	N. of subjects	References
Normal breathing	6 L/min	-	Medical textbooks
Healthy subjects	7.7 ± 0.3 L/min	19	Douglas et al, 1982
Healthy males	8.4 ± 1.3 L/min	10	Burki, 1984
Healthy males	6.3 L/min	10	Smits et al, 1987
Healthy males	6.1±1.4 L/min	6	Fuller et al, 1987
Healthy subjects	6.1± 0.9 L/min	9	Tanaka et al, 1988
Healthy students	7.0 ± 1.0 L/min	10	Turley et al, 1993
Healthy subjects	6.6 ± 0.6 L/min	10	Bengtsson et al, 1994
Healthy subjects	7.0±1.2 L/min	12	Sherman et al, 1996
Healthy subjects	7.0±1.2 L/min	10	Bell et al, 1996
Healthy subjects	6 ± 1 L/min	7	Parreira et al, 1997
Healthy subjects	7.0 ± 1.1 L/min	14	Mancini et al, 1999
Healthy subjects	6.6 ± 1.1 L/min	40	Pinna et al, 2006
Healthy subjects	6.7 ± 0.5 L/min	17	Pathak et al, 2006
Healthy subjects	6.7 ± 0.3 L/min	14	Gujic et al, 2007

Note that "healthy subjects" is not the same as "normal subjects" since ordinary modern people do not have normal breathing parameters and normal body oxygenation.

References for the Table (in the same order)

Douglas NJ, White DP, Pickett CK,l, Zwillich CW, *Respiration during sleep in normal man*, Thorax. 1982 Nov; 37(11): p.840-8Hatha Yoga Pradipika (15 century) 44.

Burki NK, *Ventilatory effects of doxapram in conscious human subjects*, Chest 1984 May; 85(5): p.600-604.

Smits P, Schouten J, Thien T, *Respiratory stimulant effects of adenosine in man after caffeine and enprofylline*, Br J Clin Pharmacol. 1987 Dec; 24(6): p.816-819.

Fuller RW, Maxwell DL, Conradson TB, Dixon CM, Barnes PJ, *Circulatory and respiratory effects of infused adenosine in conscious man*, Br J Clin Pharmacol 1987 Sep; 24(3): p.306-317.

Tanaka Y, Morikawa T, Honda Y, *An assessment of nasal functions in control of breathing*, J of Appl Physiol 1988, 65 (4); p.1520-1524.

Turley KR, McBride PJ, Wilmore LH, *Resting metabolic rate measured after subjects spent the night at home vs at a clinic*, Am J of Clin Nutr 1993, 58, p.141-144.

Bengtsson J, Bengtsson A, Stenqvist O, Bengtsson JP, *Effects of hyperventilation on the inspiratory to end- tidal oxygen difference*, British J of Anaesthesia 1994; 73: p. 140-144.

Sherman MS, Lang DM, Matityahu A, Campbell D, *Theophylline improves measurements of respiratory muscle efficiency*, Chest 1996 Dec; 110(6): p. 437-414.

Bell SC, Saunders MJ, Elborn JS, Shale DJ, *Resting energy expenditure and oxygen cost of breathing in patients with cystic fibrosis*, Thorax 1996 Feb; 51(2): 126-131.

Parreira VF, Delguste P, Jounieaux V, Aubert G, Dury M, Rodenstein DO, *Effectiveness of controlled and spontaneous modes in nasal two-level positive pressure ventilation in awake and asleep normal subjects*, Chest 1997 Nov 5; 112(5): p.1267-1277.

Mancini M, Filippelli M, Seghieri G, Iandelli I, Innocenti F, Duranti R, Scano G, *Respiratory Muscle Function and Hypoxic Ventilatory Control in Patients With Type I Diabetes*, Chest 1999; 115; p.1553-1562.

Pinna GD, Maestri R, La Rovere MT, Gobbi E, Fanfulla F, *Effect of paced breathing on ventilatory and cardiovascular variability parameters during short-term investigations of autonomic function*, Am J Physiol Heart Circ Physiol. 2006 Jan; 290(1): p.H424-433.

Pathak A, Velez-Roa S, Xhaët O, Najem B, van de Borne P, *Dose-dependent effect of dobutamine on chemoreflex activity in healthy volunteers*, Br J Clin Pharmacol. 2006 Sep; 62(3): p.272-279.

Gujic M, Houssière A, Xhaët O, Argacha JF, Denewet N, Noseda A, Jespers P, Melot C, Naeije R, van de Borne P, *Does endothelin play a role in chemoreception during acute hypoxia in normal men?* Chest. 2007 May; 131(5): p.1467-1472.

2.3 Other parameters of normal breathing

"*If a person breath-holds after a normal exhalation, it takes about 40 seconds before breathing commences*" (McArdle et al, 2000). This 40 seconds indicate normal oxygenation of cells and tissues of the human body. Note that this breath holding test is done after usual exhalation, and it does not imply any stress.

The current medical norm for CO_2 content in the alveoli of the lungs is about 40 mm Hg (or about 5.3%). End-tidal gas (at the end of the usual exhalation) and the arterial blood have nearly the same CO_2 levels or about 40 mm Hg CO_2 partial pressure. This number related to arterial CO_2 was established during the first decade of the 20th century by famous British physiologists Charles G. Douglas and John S. Haldane from Oxford University. Their results were published in 1909 article "*The regulation of normal breathing*" by the Journal of Physiology (Douglas & Haldane, 1909). This corresponds to about 5.3% (at sea level). There is no need to remember all these numbers. We need them mainly for comparisons.

Normal breathing is regular (or periodic). It is invisible (no chest or belly movements), mainly diaphragmatic, and inaudible (no panting, no wheezing, no sighing, no yawning, no sneezing, no coughing, no deep inhalations or exhalations).

Does this tiny breathing that people even do not feel provide enough oxygen for the blood? **According to numerous medical textbooks, this very small and slow normal diaphragmatic breathing** (for more information, visit http://www.normalbreathing.com/learn-8-diaphragmatic-breathing.php) **leads to nearly ideal oxygenation of the arterial blood or about 98-99%.**

Now, we can say, "Aha! Breathing more cannot increase blood and, hence, body oxygenation". This first practical conclusion is important since most yoga teachers believe in a myth that deep breathing or breathing additional air leads to increased blood oxygenation.

In reality, one can breathe 3-5, or even 10 times more than the medical norm, but blood oxygenation and delivery of oxygen to cells will not be improved to any essential degree. In fact, in real life, if we consider virtually all people with heavy breathing, their blood oxygenation becomes less. As it is easy to notice those who have heavy breathing at rest (breathing that is possible to see and hear) are chest breathers. Chest

17

breathing, by definition, does not provide fresh air for the lower parts of the lungs. The textbook, *Respiratory Physiology* (West, 2000), suggests that the lower 10% of the lungs transports more than 40 ml of oxygen per minute, while the upper 10% of the lungs transports less than 6 ml of oxygen per minute. Hence, the lower parts of the lungs are about 6-7 times more effective in oxygen transport than the top of the lungs due to richer blood supply mostly caused by gravity.

Myth: Deep breathing (for more information, visit http://www.normalbreathing.com/CO2-deep-breathing-myth.php) **or taking one or more full or maximum inhalations using the abdominal or diaphragmatic muscles increases blood and body oxygenation.**

This is just the beginning of the story related to deep breathing at rest and effects of "toxic" CO_2. However, before studying the effects of CO_2 and details of oxygen transport (and why old yoga could cure chronic diseases), I want to prove the most outrageous fact: you are very unlikely to have normal breathing. Therefore, you will discover later, using a simple DIY body oxygen test that you do not have normal body and brain oxygenation.

References

Douglas CG, Haldane JS, *The regulation of normal breathing*, Journal of Physiology 1909; 38: p. 420–440.

McArdle W.D., Katch F.I., Katch V.L., *Essentials of exercise physiology* (2-nd edition); Lippincott, Williams and Wilkins, London 2000.

West JB, *Respiratory physiology: the essentials*. 6th ed. Philadelphia: Lippincott, Williams and Wilkins; 2000.

3. You are likely a ... heavy breather

3.1 Breathing in people with heart disease

If you suffer from heart disease, you have heavy breathing 24/7 (for more information, visit http://www.normalbreathing.com/patterns-heavy-breathing.php). Here are the results of 8 published independent medical studies about breathing rates (minute ventilation) in 8 different groups of patients with heart disease. You can spot a short bar in the left bottom corner that represents normal breathing. The other bars correspond to groups of heart patients.

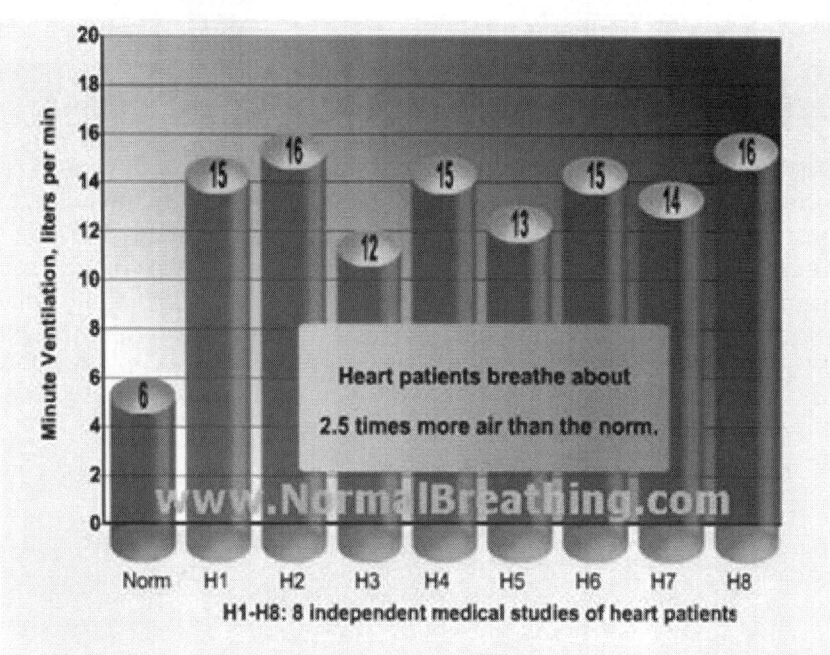

Table. Breathing rates in patients with heart disease.
*One row corresponds to one medical study/publication

Minute ventilation rates in heart patients

Condition	Minute ventilation	Number of patients	References
Normal breathing	6 L/min	-	Medical textbooks
Healthy Subjects	6-7 L/min	>400	Results of 14 studies
Heart disease	15 (±4) L/min	22	Dimopoulou et al, 2001
Heart disease	16 (±2) L/min	11	Johnson et al, 2000
Heart disease	12 (±3) L/min	132	Fanfulla et al, 1998
Heart disease	15 (±4) L/min	55	Clark et al, 1997
Heart disease	13 (±4) L/min	15	Banning et al, 1995
Heart disease	15 (±4) L/min	88	Clark et al, 1995
Heart disease	14 (±2) L/min	30	Buller et al, 1990
Heart disease	16 (±6) L/min	20	Elborn et al, 1990

Based on laws of physiology and medicine, it is possible to prove that virtually all symptoms and health problems in heart patients relate to their heavy breathing. In other words, you can have problems with heart disease only if your breathing is way heavier than the medical norm. You learn how to get back to the norm (using smart steps and correctly done yoga), all your symptoms and problems due to heart disease will disappear.

References (in the same order)

Dimopoulou I, Tsintzas OK, Alivizatos PA, Tzelepis GE, *Pattern of breathing during progressive exercise in chronic heart failure*, Int J Cardiol. 2001 Dec; 81(2-3): p. 117-121.

Johnson BD, Beck KC, Olson LJ, O'Malley KA, Allison TG, Squires RW, Gau GT, *Ventilatory constraints during exercise in patients with chronic heart failure*, Chest 2000 Feb; 117(2): p. 321-332.

Fanfulla F, Mortara , Maestri R, Pinna GD, Bruschi C, Cobelli F, Rampulla C, *The development of hyperventilation in patients with chronic heart failure and Cheyne-Stokes respiration*, Chest 1998; 114; p. 1083-1090.

Clark AL, Volterrani M, Swan JW, Coats AJS, *The increased ventilatory response to exercise in chronic heart failure: relation to pulmonary pathology*, Heart 1997; 77: p.138-146.

Banning AP, Lewis NP, Northridge DB, Elbom JS, Henderson AH, *Perfusion/ventilation mismatch during exercise in chronic heart failure: an investigation of circulatory determinants*, Br Heart J 1995; 74: p.27-33.

Clark AL, Chua TP, Coats AJ, *Anatomical dead space, ventilatory pattern, and exercise capacity in chronic heart failure*, Br Heart J 1995 Oct; 74(4): p. 377-380.

Buller NP, Poole-Wilson PA, *Mechanism of the increased ventilatory response to exercise in patients with chronic heart failure*, Heart 1990; 63; p.281-283.

Elborn JS, Riley M, Stanford CF, Nicholls DP, *The effects of flosequinan on submaximal exercise in patients with chronic cardiac failure*, Br J Clin Pharmacol. 1990 May; 29(5): p.519-524.

3.2 "Asthmatic" means a deep breather

If you do not have heart disease, then you may have asthma (for more information, visit http://www.normalbreathing.com/diseases-Asthma.php). Let us look at MV (minute ventilation) in patients with asthma when they are at rest. Here again, the breathing rates relate to the state of patients when they do not have any acute episodes or symptoms of their disease, since during exacerbations, chronically sick people breathe even more.

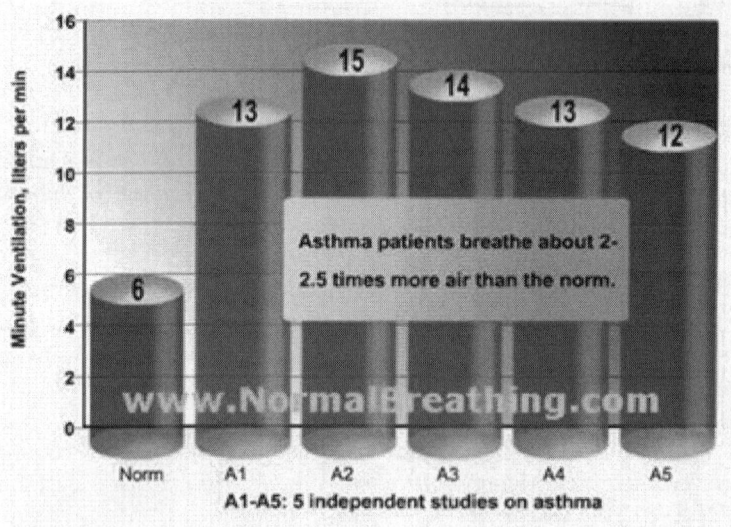

Table. Breathing rates in people with asthma.
*One row corresponds to one medical study/publication

Minute ventilation rates in asthmatics

Condition	Minute ventilation	Number of people	References
Normal breathing	6 L/min	-	Medical textbooks
Healthy Subjects	6-7 L/min	>400	Results of 14 studies
Asthma	13 (±2) L/min	16	Chalupa et al, 2004
Asthma	15 L/min	8	Johnson et al, 1995
Asthma	14 (±6) L/min	39	Bowler et al, 1998
Asthma	13 (±4) L/min	17	Kassabian et al, 1982
Asthma	12 L/min	101	McFadden & Lyons, 1968

References (in the same order)

Chalupa DC, Morrow PE, Oberdörster G, Utell MJ, Frampton MW, *Ultrafine particle deposition in subjects with asthma*, Environmental Health Perspectives 2004 Jun; 112(8): p.879-882.

Johnson BD, Scanlon PD, Beck KC, *Regulation of ventilatory capacity during exercise in asthmatics*, J Appl Physiol. 1995 Sep; 79(3): 892-901.

Bowler SD, Green A, Mitchell CA, *Buteyko breathing techniques in asthma: a blinded randomised controlled trial*, Med J of Australia 1998; 169: 575-578.

Kassabian J, Miller KD, Lavietes MH, *Respiratory center output and ventilatory timing in patients with acute airway (asthma) and alveolar (pneumonia) disease*, Chest 1982 May; 81(5): p.536-543.

McFadden ER & Lyons HA, *Arterial-blood gases in asthma*, The New Engl J of Med 1968 May 9, 278 (19): 1027-1032.

3.3 Deep breathing in people with diabetes

If you do not have asthma or heart disease, then you may suffer from diabetes (for more information, visit http://www.normalbreathing.com/c/diabetes.php). Diabetes means deep breathing 24/7, because if a diabetic achieves normal breathing parameters, his or her symptoms of diabetes and abnormal blood sugar levels will disappear.

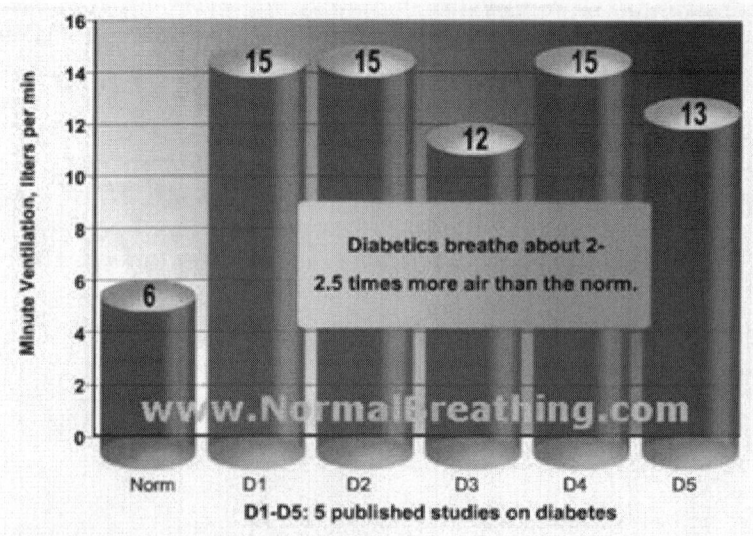

Table. Breathing rates in diabetics.
*One row corresponds to one medical study/publication

Minute ventilation rates in diabetics

Condition	Minute ventilation	Number of people	References
Normal breathing	6 L/min	-	Medical textbooks
Healthy Subjects	6-7 L/min	>400	Results of 14 studies
Diabetes	12-17 L/min	26	Bottini et al, 2003
Diabetes	15 (±2) L/min	45	Tantucci et al, 2001
Diabetes	12 (±2) L/min	8	Mancini et al, 1999
Diabetes	10-20 L/min	28	Tantucci et al, 1997
Diabetes	13 (±2) L/min	20	Tantucci et al, 1996

References (in the same order)

Bottini P, Dottorini ML, M. Cordoni MC, Casucci G, Tantucci C, *Sleep-disordered breathing in nonobese diabetic subjects with autonomic neuropathy*, Eur Respir J 2003; 22: p. 654–660.

Tantucci C, Bottini P, Fiorani C, Dottorini ML, Santeusanio F, Provinciali L, Sorbini CA, Casucci G, *Cerebrovascular reactivity and hypercapnic respiratory drive in diabetic autonomic neuropathy*, J Appl Physiol 2001, 90: p. 889–896.

Mancini M, Filippelli M, Seghieri G, Iandelli I, Innocenti F, Duranti R, Scano G, *Respiratory Muscle Function and Hypoxic Ventilatory Control in Patients With Type I Diabetes*, Chest 1999; 115; p.1553-1562.

Tantucci C, Scionti L, Bottini P, Dottorini ML, Puxeddu E, Casucci G, Sorbini CA, *Influence of autonomic neuropathy of different severities on the hypercapnic drive to breathing in diabetic patients*, Chest. 1997 Jul; 112(1): p. 145-153.

Tantucci C, Bottini P, Dottorini ML, Puxeddu E, Casucci G, Scionti L, Sorbini CA, *Ventilatory response to exercise in diabetic subjects with autonomic neuropathy*, J Appl Physiol 1996, 81(5): p.1978–1986.

3.4 People with other chronic diseases are also heavy breathers

Even if you are from those 3 diseases, you can have some others. The following studies also show that heavy or deep breathing is a norm in people with cancer, COPD, liver cirrhosis, epilepsy, cystic fibrosis, panic disorder, bipolar disorder, etc.

Table. Minute ventilation in patients with other chronic conditions.
*One row corresponds to one medical study/publication

Condition	Minute ventilation	Number of people	References
Normal breathing	6 L/min	-	Medical textbooks
Healthy Subjects	6-7 L/min	>400	Results of 14 studies
Pulm hypertension	12 (±2) L/min	11	D'Alonzo et al, 1987
Cancer	12 (±2) L/min	40	Travers et al, 2008
COPD	14 (±2) L/min	12	Palange et al, 2001
COPD	12 (±2) L/min	10	Sinderby et al, 2001
COPD	14 L/min	3	Stulbarg et al, 2001
Sleep apnea	15 (±3) L/min	20	Radwan et al, 2001
Liver cirrhosis	11-18 L/min	24	Epstein et al, 1998
Hyperthyroidism	15 (±1) L/min	42	Kahaly, 1998
Cystic fibrosis	15 L/min	15	Fauroux et al, 2006
Cystic fibrosis	10 L/min	11	Browning et al, 1990
Cystic fibrosis*	10 L/min	10	Ward et al, 1999
CF and diabetes*	10 L/min	7	Ward et al, 1999
Cystic fibrosis	16 L/min	7	Dodd et al, 2006
Cystic fibrosis	18 L/min	9	McKone et al, 2005
Cystic fibrosis*	13 (±2) L/min	10	Bell et al, 1996
Cystic fibrosis	11-14 L/min	6	Tepper et al, 1983
Epilepsy	13 L/min	12	Esquivel et al, 1991
CHV	13 (±2) L/min	134	Han et al, 1997
Panic disorder	12 (±5) L/min	12	Pain et al, 1991
Bipolar disorder	11 (±2) L/min	16	MacKinnon et al, 2007
Dystrophia myotonica	16 (±4) L/min	12	Clague et al, 1994

There are many more published studies that demonstrated the same results: **Sick people have a deep or heavy breathing pattern at rest.** In fact, all of the studies which I have found online and libraries demonstrated the same conclusion: sick people breathe too much air in comparison with the medical norm.

Even if you do not suffer from these health problems, I am still going to prove in the next section that you also "follow" the advice of modern yoga teachers to breathe too much air. I will also show that your overbreathing is the cause of your current health problems.

References (in the same order)

D'Alonzo GE, Gianotti LA, Pohil RL, Reagle RR, DuRee SL, Fuentes F, Dantzker DR, *Comparison of progressive exercise performance of normal subjects and patients with primary pulmonary hypertension*, Chest 1987 Jul; 92(1): p.57-62.

Travers J, Dudgeon DJ, Amjadi K, McBride I, Dillon K, Laveneziana P, Ofir D, Webb KA, O'Donnell DE, *Mechanisms of exertional dyspnea in patients with cancer*, J Appl Physiol 2008 Jan; 104(1): p.57-66.

Palange P, Valli G, Onorati P, Antonucci R, Paoletti P, Rosato A, Manfredi F, Serra P, *Effect of heliox on lung dynamic hyperinflation, dyspnea, and exercise endurance capacity in COPD patients*, J Appl Physiol. 2004 Nov; 97(5): p.1637-1642.

Sinderby C, Spahija J, Beck J, Kaminski D, Yan S, Comtois N, Sliwinski P, *Diaphragm activation during exercise in chronic obstructive pulmonary disease*, Am J Respir Crit Care Med 2001 Jun; 163(7): 1637-1641.

Stulbarg MS, Winn WR, Kellett LE, *Bilateral Carotid Body Resection for the Relief of Dyspnea in Severe Chronic Obstructive Pulmonary Disease*, Chest 1989; 95 (5): p.1123-1128.

Radwan L, Maszczyk Z, Koziorowski A, Koziej M, Cieslicki J, Sliwinski P, Zielinski J, *Control of breathing in obstructive sleep apnoea and in patients with the overlap syndrome*, Eur Respir J. 1995 Apr; 8(4): p.542-545.

Epstein SK, Zilberberg MD; Facoby C, Ciubotaru RL, Kaplan LM, *Response to symptom-limited exercise in patients with the hepatopulmonary syndrome*, Chest 1998; 114; p. 736-741.

Kahaly GJ, Nieswandt J, Wagner S, Schlegel J, Mohr-Kahaly S, Hommel G, *Ineffective cardiorespiratory function in hyperthyroidism*, J Clin Endocrinol Metab 1998 Nov; 83(11): p. 4075-4078.

Fauroux B, Nicot F, Boelle PY, Boulé M, Clément A, Lofaso F, Bonora M, *Mechanical limitation during CO2 rebreathing in young patients with cystic fibrosis*, Respir Physiol Neurobiol. 2006 Oct 27;153(3):217-25. Epub 2005 Dec 27.

Browning IB, D'Alonzo GE, Tobin MJ, *Importance of respiratory rate as an indicator of respiratory dysfunction in patients with cystic fibrosis*, Chest. 1990 Jun;97(6):1317-21.

Ward SA, Tomezsko JL, Holsclaw DS, Paolone AM, *Energy expenditure and substrate utilization in adults with cystic fibrosis and diabetes mellitus*, Am J Clin Nutr. 1999 May;69(5):913-9.

Dodd JD, Barry SC, Barry RB, Gallagher CG, Skehan SJ, Masterson JB, *Thin-section CT in patients with cystic fibrosis: correlation with peak exercise capacity and body mass index*, Radiology. 2006 Jul;240(1):236-45.

McKone EF, Barry SC, Fitzgerald MX, Gallagher CG, *Role of arterial hypoxemia and pulmonary mechanics in exercise limitation in adults with cystic fibrosis*, J Appl Physiol. 2005 Sep;99(3):1012-8.

Bell SC, Saunders MJ, Elborn JS, Shale DJ, *Resting energy expenditure and oxygen cost of breathing in patients with cystic fibrosis*, Thorax 1996 Feb; 51(2): 126-131.

Tepper RS, Skatrud B, Dempsey JA, *Ventilation and oxygenation changes during sleep in cystic fibrosis*, Chest 1983; 84; p. 388-393.

Esquivel E, Chaussain M, Plouin P, Ponsot G, Arthuis M, *Physical exercise and voluntary hyperventilation in childhood absence epilepsy*, Electroencephalogr Clin Neurophysiol 1991 Aug; 79(2): p. 127-132.

Han JN, Stegen K, Simkens K, Cauberghs M, Schepers R, Van den Bergh O, Clément J, Van de Woestijne KP, *Unsteadiness of breathing in patients with hyperventilation syndrome and anxiety disorders*, Eur Respir J 1997; 10: p. 167–176.

Pain MC, Biddle N, Tiller JW, *Panic disorder, the ventilatory response to carbon dioxide and respiratory variables*, Psychosom Med 1988 Sep-Oct; 50(5): p. 541-548.

MacKinnon DF, Craighead B, Hoehn-Saric R, *Carbon dioxide provocation of anxiety and respiratory response in bipolar disorder*, J Affect Disord 2007 Apr; 99(1-3): p.45-49.

Clague JE, Carter J, Coakley J, Edwards RH, Calverley PM, *Respiratory effort perception at rest and during carbon dioxide rebreathing in patients with dystrophia myotonica*, Thorax 1994 Mar; 49(3): p.240-244.

3.5 Over 90% of modern people, you probably included, breathe too much air

Finally, if you avoided all those health problems that are considered above, you are still likely be the person who has heavy breathing days and nights. Here are hard medical facts.

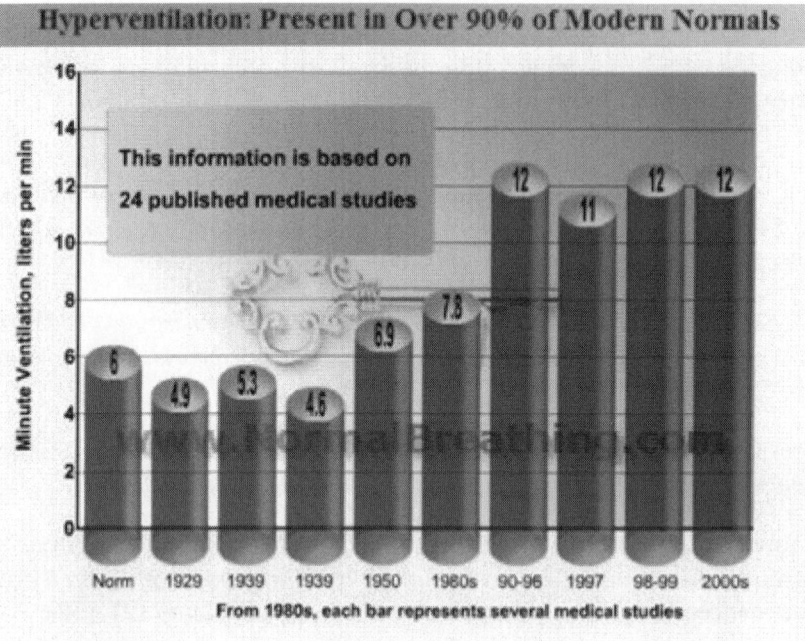

Yoga Benefits are in Breathing Less — Artour Rakhimov

The table below represents results of 24 medical research studies (from 1929 until year 2007). It tells us that before WW2 breathing rates of ordinary people were even less than normal. During last 2 decades ordinary people breathe about 2 times more air than the medical norm or nearly 3 times more than in the 1920's and 30's.

Table. Historical changes in minute ventilation at rest for normal subjects

Condition	Minute ventilation	Age	N. of subjects	References
Healthy Subjects	6-7 L/min	-	>400	Results of 14 studies
Normal breathing	6	-	-	Medical textbooks
Normal subjects	4.9	-	5	Griffith et al, 1929
Normal males	5.3±0.1	27-43	46	Shock et al, 1939
Normal females	4.6±0.1	27-43	40	Shock et al, 1939
Normal subjects	6.9±0.9	-	100	Matheson et al, 1950
Normal subjects	9.1±4.5	31±7	11	Kassabian et al, 1982
Normal subjects	8.1±2.1	42±14	11	D'Alonzo et al, 1987
Normal subjects	6.3±2.2	-	12	Pain et al, 1988
Normal males	13±3	40 (av.)	12	Clague et al, 1994
Normal subjects	9.2±2.5	34±7	13	Radwan et al, 1995
Normal subjects	15±4	28-34	12	Dahan et al, 1995
Normal subjects	12±4	55±10	43	Clark et al, 1995
Normal subjects	12±2	41±2	10	Tantucci et al, 1996
Normal subjects*	11±3	53±11	24	Clark et al, 1997

(table continues on next page)

Table. Historical changes in minute ventilation at rest for normal subjects (cont'd)

Normal subjects	8.1±0.4	34±2	63	Meessen et al, 1997
Normal females	9.9	20-28	23	Han et al, 1997
Normal males	15	20-28	47	Han et al, 1997
Normal females	10	29-60	42	Han et al, 1997
Normal males	11	29-62	42	Han et al, 1997
Normal subjects	13±3	36±6	10	Tantucci et al, 1997
Normal subjects	12±1	65±2	10	Epstein et al, 1996
Normal subjects	12±1	12-69	20	Bowler et al, 1998
Normal subjects	10±6	39±4	20	DeLorey et al, 1999
Normal seniors	12±4	70±3	14	DeLorey et al, 1999
Normal elderly*	14±3	88±2	11	DeLorey et al, 1999
Normal subjects	17±1	41±2	15	Tantucci et al, 2001
Normal subjects	10±0.5	-	10	Bell et al, 2005
Normal subjects	8.5±1.2	30±8	69	Narkiewicz, 2006
Normal females	10±0.4	-	11	Ahuja et al, 2007
Normal subjects	12±2	62±2	20	Travers et al, 2008
Condition	Minute ventilation	Age	N. of subjects	Reference

* When the average weight of the subjects was significantly different from 70 kg, minute ventilation was adjusted to the normal weight (70 kg) value.

Note that the results look inconsistent since there is no strict definition for "normal" or "control" subjects in medical research. In addition, there are slightly different methods used to measure minute ventilation. Consider a medical study with a group of people with heart disease. If the organizers of the study want to see the effects of some medication or treatment method for these people with heart disease, the researchers may also select a group of control subjects for comparison (the control group). For some studies they require that these "control" subjects are free from any form of heart disease. However, in other studies, the control subjects should be free from any health problem. Then they can be called "healthy subjects".

Now we are going to prove that breathing (for more information, visit http://www.normalbreathing.com) more reduces brain and body oxygen content. Later, we are going to discuss the DIY test that accurately reflects body O2 content.

References for the Table (in the same order)

Griffith FR, Pucher GW, Brownell KA, Klein JD, Carmer ME, *Studies in human physiology. IV. Vital capacity, respiratory rate and volume, and composition of the expired air*. Am. J. Physiol 1929, vol. 89, p. 555.

Shock NW, Soley MH, *Average Values for Basal Respiratory Functions in Adolescents and Adults*, J. Nutrition, 1939, 18, p. 143.

Matheson HW, Gray JS, V*entilatory function tests. III Resting ventilation, metabolism, and derived measures*, J Clin Invest 1950 June; 29(6): p. 688–692.

Kassabian J, Miller KD, Lavietes MH, *Respiratory center output and ventilatory timing in patients with acute airway (asthma) and alveolar (pneumonia) disease*, Chest 1982 May; 81(5): p.536-543.

D'Alonzo GE, Gianotti LA, Pohil RL, Reagle RR, DuRee SL, Fuentes F, Dantzker DR, *Comparison of progressive exercise performance of normal subjects and patients with primary pulmonary hypertension*, Chest 1987 Jul; 92(1): p.57-62.

Pain MC, Biddle N, Tiller JW, *Panic disorder, the ventilatory response to carbon dioxide and respiratory variables*, Psychosom Med 1988 Sep-Oct; 50(5): p. 541-548.

Clague JE, Carter J, Coakley J, Edwards RH, Calverley PM, *Respiratory effort perception at rest and during carbon dioxide rebreathing in patients with dystrophia myotonica*, Thorax 1994 Mar; 49(3): p.240-244.

Radwan L, Maszczyk Z, Koziorowski A, Koziej M, Cieslicki J, Sliwinski P, Zielinski J, *Control of breathing in obstructive sleep apnoea and in patients with the overlap syndrome*, Eur Respir J. 1995 Apr; 8(4): p.542-545.

Dahan A, van den Elsen MJ, Berkenbosch A, DeGoede J, Olievier IC, van Kleef JW, *Halothane affects ventilatory afterdischarge in humans*, Br J Anaesth 1995 May; 74(5): p.544-548.

Clark AL, Chua TP, Coats AJ, *Anatomical dead space, ventilatory pattern, and exercise capacity in chronic heart failure*, Br Heart J 1995 Oct; 74(4): p. 377-380.

Tantucci C, Bottini P, Dottorini ML, Puxeddu E, Casucci G, Scionti L, Sorbini CA, *Ventilatory response to exercise in diabetic subjects with autonomic neuropathy*, J Appl Physiol 1996, 81(5): p.1978–1986.

Clark AL, Volterrani M, Swan JW, Coats AJS, *The increased ventilatory response to exercise in chronic heart failure: relation to pulmonary pathology*, Heart 1997; 77: p.138-146.

Meessen NE, van der Grinten CP, Luijendijk SC, Folgering HT, *Breathing pattern during bronchial challenge in humans*, Eur Respir J 1997 May; 10(5): p.1059-1063.

Han JN, Stegen K, Simkens K, Cauberghs M, Schepers R, Van den Bergh O, Clément J, Van de Woestijne KP, *Unsteadiness of breathing in patients with hyperventilation syndrome and anxiety disorders*, Eur Respir J 1997; 10: p. 167–176.

Tantucci C, Scionti L, Bottini P, Dottorini ML, Puxeddu E, Casucci G, Sorbini CA, *Influence of autonomic neuropathy of different severities on the hypercapnic drive to breathing in diabetic patients*, Chest. 1997 Jul; 112(1): 145-153.

Epstein SK, Zilberberg MD; Facoby C, Ciubotaru RL, Kaplan LM, *Response to symptom-limited exercise in patients with the hepatopulmonary syndrome*, Chest 1998; 114; p. 736-741.

Bowler SD, Green A, Mitchell CA, *Buteyko breathing techniques in asthma: a blinded randomised controlled trial*, Med J of Australia 1998; 169: p. 575-578.

DeLorey DS, Babb TG, *Progressive mechanical ventilatory constraints with aging*, Am J Respir Crit Care Med 1999 Jul; 160(1): p.169-177.

Tantucci C, Bottini P, Fiorani C, Dottorini ML, Santeusanio F, Provinciali L, Sorbini CA, Casucci G, *Cerebrovascular reactivity and hypercapnic respiratory drive in diabetic autonomic neuropathy*, J Appl Physiol 2001, 90: p. 889–896.

Bell HJ, Feenstra W, Duffin J, *The initial phase of exercise hyperpnoea in humans is depressed during a cognitive task*, Experimental Physiology 2005 May; 90(3): p.357-365.

Narkiewicz K, van de Borne P, Montano N, Hering D, Kara T, Somers VK, *Sympathetic neural outflow and chemoreflex sensitivity are related to spontaneous breathing rate in normal men*, Hypertension 2006 Jan; 47(1): p.51-55.

Ahuja D, Mateika JH, Diamond MP, Badr MS, *Ventilatory sensitivity to carbon dioxide before and after episodic hypoxia in women treated with testosterone*, J Appl Physiol. 2007 May; 102(5): p.1832-1838.

Travers J, Dudgeon DJ, Amjadi K, McBride I, Dillon K, Laveneziana P, Ofir D, Webb KA, O'Donnell DE, *Mechanisms of exertional dyspnea in patients with cancer*, J Appl Physiol 2008 Jan; 104(1): p.57-66.

4. Effects of deep breathing (hyperventilation)

We proved that you have heavy breathing at rest in spite of your possible love for yoga and hundreds or thousands of yoga lessons that you practiced. Now we are going to study the effects of your heavy breathing (hyperventilation) (for more information, visit http://www.normalbreathing.com/i-hyperventilation.php) on body oxygenation, states of your brain and other systems and organs.

4.1 Hypocapnia (or CO2 deficiency in the blood and cells)

If a healthy or ordinary person starts to breathe more air (or deeper and/or faster), what are the effects?

- More carbon dioxide is removed from the lungs with every breath and therefore the level of CO2 in the alveoli of the lungs immediately decreases
- In 1-2 minutes of overbreathing, the arterial CO2 level falls below the normal levels in all the arterial blood due to its circulation
  In 3-5 minutes, due to CO2 diffusion from cells and tissues, most cells of the body (including the cells of the heart, kidneys, liver, pancreas, stomach, muscle tissues and many others) experience lowered CO2 concentrations
- In 15-20 minutes, the CO2 level in the cerebrospinal fluid of the brain also drops below the norm due to a slower diffusion rate through the blood-brain barrier.

* Note. There is a small group of people who suffer from severe problems with their lungs. This relates to people who have emphysema, severe asthma, severe bronchitis, lung cancer, and some other conditions. These people do not get low CO2 in the blood, brain and other body cells. However, their problems with lungs will cause the same

key final effect: low O2 in body cells. In fact, their hypoxia is usually the most severe one since they are the first candidates for supplemental oxygen (breathing 100% oxygen that is toxic). I can only add that their heavy breathing destroys their lungs and worsens their health. It is beyond the scope of this book to focus on further details related to such cases.

4.2 Vasoconstriction

Does CO2 produce any effects on blood vessels? Yes, as independent physiological studies found, hypocapnia (low CO2 concentration in the arterial blood) decreases perfusion of the following organs:

- brain (Fortune et al, 1995; Karlsson et al, 1994; Liem et al, 1995; Macey et al, 2007; Santiago & Edelman, 1986; Starling & Evans, 1968; Tsuda et al, 1987)
- heart (Coetzee et al, 1984; Foëx et al, 1979; Karlsson et al, 1994; Okazaki et al, 1991; Okazaki et al, 1992; Wexels et al, 1985)
- liver (Dutton et al, 1976; Fujita et al, 1989; Hughes et al, 1979; Okazaki, 1989)
- kidneys (Karlsson et al, 1994; Okazaki, 1989)
- spleen (Karlsson et al, 1994)
- colon (Gilmour et al, 1980).

What is the physiological mechanism of the reduced blood flow to vital organs? CO2 is a dilator of blood vessels (arteries and arterioles) or a vasodilator. Arteries and arterioles have their own tiny smooth muscles that can constrict or dilate depending on CO2 concentrations. When we breathe more, CO2 level in the arterial blood decreases, blood vessels constrict and vital organs (like the brain, heart, kidneys, liver, stomach, spleen, colon, etc.) get less blood supply.

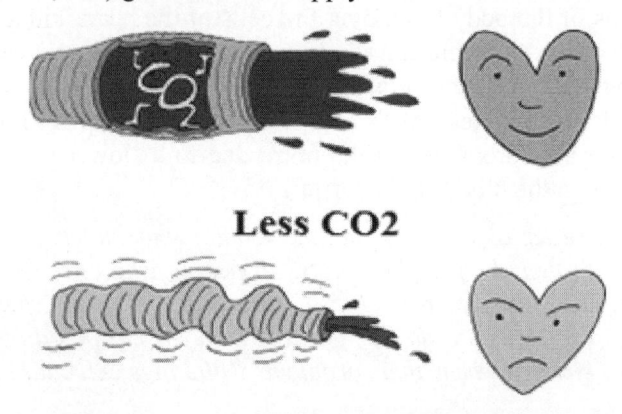

Less CO2

Yoga Benefits are in Breathing Less — Artour Rakhimov

There are literally hundreds of studies that proved or showed presence of this vasoconstriction (for more information, visit http://www.normalbreathing.com/CO2-vasodilation.php) effect. Some people may argue that this is just a small or insignificant effect, and there are more powerful vasodilators. According to Dr. M. Kashiba, MD and his medical colleagues from the Department of Biochemistry and Integrative Medical Biology (School of Medicine, Keio University, Tokyo, Japan) CO2 is a "*potent vasodilator*" (Kashiba et al, 2002). Dr. H. G. Djurberg and his medical team from the Department of Anesthesia (Armed Forces Hospital, Riyadh, Saudi Arabia) suggested that "*Carbon dioxide, a most potent cerebral vasodilator...*" (Djurberg et al, 1998). Among arterial dilators, CO2 is probably the most powerful chemical. This vasodilation effect is present in healthy people due to normal arterial CO2 concentration.

If a yoga student follows the ideas about breathing more ("to get more oxygen in body cells") and expel toxic CO2, such yoga practice will lead to spasm of all arteries and arterioles and reduced circulation to all vital organs. The effects of overbreathing are individual. There are certain individual short-term effects (like the one described by Bikram Choudhury above) and numerous long-term effects that relate to chronic diseases. Note that if one practices deep breathing exercises with CO2 losses, then this practice leads to deeper and faster breathing for many subsequent hours because breathing is controlled mainly by CO2 and low CO2 means heavy automatic breathing later.

Are there any related systemic effects due to vasoconstriction? The state of these blood vessels (arteries and arterioles) defines the total resistance to the systemic blood flow in the human body since these blood vessels provide the main resistance to blood flow. Hence, hypocapnia or low CO2 constricts the most important blood vessels and increases the strain on the heart. Hence, in a long run, automatic breathing directly participates in regulation of the heart rate. The father of cardiorespiratory physiology, Yale University Professor Yandell Henderson (1873-1944), investigated this effect more than a century ago.

Among his numerous physiological studies, he performed clinical studies with anaesthetized dogs on mechanical ventilation. The results of these studies were described in his article "*Acapnia and shock. - I. Carbon dioxide as a factor in the regulation of the heart rate*". In this article, published in 1908 in the *American Journal of Physiology*, he wrote, "*... we were enabled to regulate the heart to any desired rate from 40 or fewer up to 200 or more beats per minute. The method was very simple.*

It depended on the manipulation of the hand bellows with which artificial respiration was administered... As the pulmonary ventilation increased or diminished the heart rate was correspondingly accelerated or retarded" (p.127, Henderson, 1908).

Symptoms due to voluntary hyperventilation

Imagine that a person at rest starts to voluntarily breathe deeply or hyperventilate (deep and fast breathing). What would happen with him or her? The person would feel dizzy and could faint or pass out. Why? This is cannot be due to too much oxygen, since their blood is almost fully saturated with O2 with very small normal breathing at rest. The key effect of vasoconstriction that reduced blood flow to the brain. This graph below is a PET scan that shows brain O2 concentrations in two conditions: normal breathing (the left image) and after 1 minute of hyperventilation (the right image). The red color (they are the small spots surrounded by lighter colors) represents the most O2, dark blue (larger darker blobs) the least, according to the scale given below the images. Overbreathing reduces brain oxygenation by about 40% or almost 2 times (Litchfield, 2003).

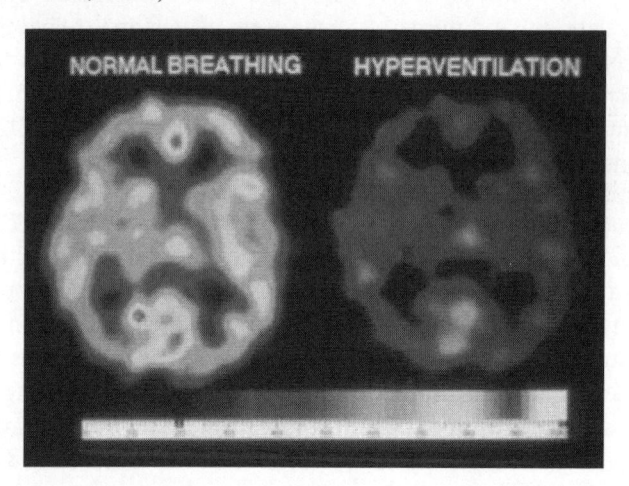

This result is also quoted in many medical textbooks (e.g., Starling & Evans, 1968) since the effect is well documented and has been confirmed by dozens of professional experiments. According to the Handbook of Physiology (Santiago & Edelman, 1986), cerebral blood flow decreases 2% for every mm Hg decrease in CO2 pressure. This means that if you reduce your arterial CO2 two times below the norm (by expelling toxic CO2). you will get twice less oxygen and blood supply provided for the brain at rest.

References

Coetzee A, Holland D, Foëx P, Ryder A, Jones L, *The effect of hypocapnia on coronary blood flow and myocardial function in the dog*, Anesthesia and Analgesia 1984 Nov; 63(11): p. 991-997.

Dutton R, Levitzky M, Berkman R, *Carbon dioxide and liver blood flow*, Bull Eur Physiopathol Respir. 1976 Mar-Apr; 12(2): p. 265-273.

Gilmour DG, Douglas IH, Aitkenhead AR, Hothersall AP, Horton PW, Ledingham IM, *Colon blood flow in the dog: effects of changes in arterial carbon dioxide tension*, Cardiovasc Res 1980 Jan; 14(1): 11-20.

Foëx P, Ryder WA, *Effect of CO2 on the systemic and coronary circulations and on coronary sinus blood gas tensions*, Bull Eur Physiopathol Respir 1979 Jul-Aug; 15(4): p.625-638.

Fortune JB, Feustel PJ, deLuna C, Graca L, Hasselbarth J, Kupinski AM, *Cerebral blood flow and blood volume in response to O2 and CO2 changes in normal humans*, J Trauma. 1995 Sep; 39(3): p. 463-471.

Fujita Y, Sakai T, Ohsumi A, Takaori M, *Effects of hypocapnia and hypercapnia on splanchnic circulation and hepatic function in the beagle*, Anesthesia and Analgesia 1989 Aug; 69(2): p. 152-157.

Hashimoto K, Okazaki K, Okutsu Y, *The effects of hypocapnia and hypercapnia on tissue surface PO2 in hemorrhaged dogs* [Article in Japanese], Masui 1989 Oct; 38(10): p. 1271-1274.

Henderson Y, *Acapnia and shock. - I. Carbon dioxide as a factor in the regulation of the heart rate*, American Journal of Physiology 1908, 21: p. 126-156.

Hughes RL, Mathie RT, Fitch W, Campbell D, *Liver blood flow and oxygen consumption during hypocapnia and IPPV in the greyhound*, J Appl Physiol. 1979 Aug; 47(2): p. 290-295.

Karlsson T, Stjernström EL, Stjernström H, Norlén K, Wiklund L, *Central and regional blood flow during hyperventilation. An experimental study in the pig*, Acta Anaesthesiol Scand. 1994 Feb; 38(2): p.180-186.

Liem KD, Kollée LA, Hopman JC, De Haan AF, Oeseburg B, *The influence of arterial carbon dioxide on cerebral oxygenation and haemodynamics during ECMO in normoxaemic and hypoxaemic piglets*, Acta Anaesthesiol Scand Suppl. 1995; 107: p.157-164.

Litchfield PM, *A brief overview of the chemistry of respiration and the breathing heart wave*, California Biofeedback, 2003 Spring, 19(1).

Macey PM, Woo MA, Harper RM, *Hyperoxic brain effects are normalized by addition of CO2*, PLoS Med. 2007 May; 4(5): p. e173.

McArdle WD, Katch FI, Katch VL, *Essentials of exercise physiology* (2-nd edition); Lippincott, Williams and Wilkins, London 2000.

Okazaki K, Okutsu Y, Fukunaga A, *Effect of carbon dioxide (hypocapnia and hypercapnia) on tissue blood flow and oxygenation of liver, kidneys and skeletal muscle in the dog*, Masui 1989 Apr, 38 (4): p. 457-464.

Okazaki K, Hashimoto K, Okutsu Y, Okumura F, *Effect of arterial carbon dioxide tension on regional myocardial tissue oxygen tension in the dog* [Article in Japanese], Masui 1991 Nov; 40(11): p. 1620-1624.

Okazaki K, Hashimoto K, Okutsu Y, Okumura F, *Effect of carbon dioxide (hypocapnia and hypercapnia) on regional myocardial tissue oxygen tension in dogs with coronary stenosis* [Article in Japanese], Masui 1992 Feb; 41(2): p. 221-224.

Santiago TV & Edelman NH, *Brain blood flow and control of breathing*, in *Handbook of Physiology, Section 3: The respiratory system*, vol. II, ed. by AP Fishman. American Physiological Society, Betheda, Maryland, 1986, p. 163-179.

Starling E & Lovatt EC, *Principles of human physiology*, 14-th ed., 1968, Lea & Febiger, Philadelphia.

Tsuda Y, Kimura K, Yoneda S, Hartmann A, Etani H, Hashikawa K, Kamada T, *Effect of hypocapnia on cerebral oxygen metabolism and blood flow in ischemic cerebrovascular disorders*, Eur Neurol. 1987; 27(3): p.155-163.

Wexels JC, Myhre ES, Mjøs OD, *Effects of carbon dioxide and pH on myocardial blood-flow and metabolism in the dog*, Clin Physiol. 1985 Dec; 5(6): p.575-588.

4.3 Suppressed Bohr effect

This is not the end of the oxygen and CO2 story since oxygen must be somehow released be red blood cells in tissues. Oxygen is a highly reactive and toxic chemical. Therefore, there is a chemical connection between oxygen molecule and the red blood cell that can carry up to 4 oxygen molecules. This chemical link that prevents oxygen from destroying walls of the blood vessels is also called "chemical affinity".

Why do red blood cells or hemoglobin cells of the arterial blood release oxygen in the tissues, but not in the arteries, or arterioles, or veins, or somewhere else? Why is more oxygen released in those tissues of the human body that produce more energy? For example, those muscles that generate more energy are going to get more oxygen from the blood. Why?

This process of oxygen release depends primarily on local CO2 content (or CO2 levels in tissues) due to the so called **Bohr law** (or **Bohr effect**)(for more information, visit http://www.normalbreathing.com/CO2-bohr-effect.php). The effect was first described in 1904 by the Danish physiologist Christian Bohr (father of famous physicist Niels Bohr). He found that due to higher CO2 concentrations in tissues (and more acidic environment), hemoglobin will bind to oxygen with less affinity. In other words, increased CO2 levels in tissues allow red blood cells to release oxygen. As a result, those tissues that generate more CO2 will get more oxygen from the blood.

There are many modern professional studies devoted to various aspects of this effect (for example, Braumann et al, 1982; Böning et al, 1975; Bucci et al, 1985; Carter et al, 1985; diBella et al, 1986; Dzhagarov et al, 1996; Grant et al, 1982; Grubb et al, 1979; Gersonde et al, 1986; Hlastala & Woodson, 1983; Jensen, 2004; Kister et al, 1988; Kobayashi et al, 1989; Lapennas, 1983; Matthew et al, 1979; Meyer et al, 1978; Tyuma, 1984; Winslow et al, 1985).

Hyperventilation and reduced CO2 tissue tension lead to hampered or reduced oxygen release and low O2 tension in tissues (Aarnoudse et al, 1981; Monday & Tétreault, 1980; Gottstein et al, 1976). In order to improve the release of oxygen by red blood cells, we require more CO2 in the cells and the whole body.

Hence, if yoga student wants to provide more oxygen for the brain, heart and other cells of the body, he or she should learn how to breathe slower and less.

References

Aarnoudse JG, Oeseburg B, Kwant G, Zwart A, Zijlstra WG, Huisjes HJ, *Influence of variations in pH and PCO2 on scalp tissue oxygen tension and carotid arterial oxygen tension in the fetal lamb*, Biol Neonate 1981; 40(5-6): p. 252-263.

Braumann KM, Böning D, Trost F, *Bohr effect and slope of the oxygen dissociation curve after physical training*, J Appl Physiol. 1982 Jun; 52(6): p. 1524-1529.

Böning D, Schwiegart U, Tibes U, Hemmer B, *Influences of exercise and endurance training on the oxygen dissociation curve of blood under in vivo and in vitro conditions*, Eur J Appl Physiol Occup Physiol. 1975; 34(1): p. 1-10.

Bucci E, Fronticelli C, *Anion Bohr effect of human hemoglobin*, Biochemistry. 1985 Jan 15; 24(2): p. 371-376.

Carter AM, Grønlund J, *Contribution of the Bohr effect to the fall in fetal PO2 caused by maternal alkalosis*, J Perinat Med. 1985; 13(4): p.185-191.

diBella G, Scandariato G, Suriano O, Rizzo A, *Oxygen affinity and Bohr effect responses to 2,3- diphosphoglycerate in equine and human blood*, Res Vet Sci. 1996 May; 60(3): p. 272-275.

Dzhagarov BM, Kruk NN, *The alkaline Bohr effect: regulation of hemoglobin Hb(O2)3* [Article in Russian] Biofizika. 1996 May-Jun; 41(3): p. 606-612.

Gersonde K, Sick H, Overkamp M, Smith KM, Parish DW, *Bohr effect in monomeric insect haemoglobins controlled by O2 off-rate and modulated by haem-rotational disorder*, Eur J Biochem. 1986 Jun 2; 157(2): p. 393-404.

Grant BJ, *Influence of Bohr-Haldane effect on steady-state gas exchange*, J Appl Physiol. 1982 May; 52(5): p. 1330-1337.

Grubb B, Jones JH, Schmidt-Nielsen K, *Avian cerebral blood flow: influence of the Bohr effect on oxygen supply*, Am J Physiol. 1979 May; 236(5): p. H744-749.

Gottstein U, Zahn U, Held K, Gabriel FH, Textor T, Berghoff W, *Effect of hyperventilation on cerebral blood flow and metabolism in man; continuous monitoring of arterio-cerebral venous glucose differences* (author's transl) [Article in German], Klin Wochenschr. 1976 Apr 15; 54(8): p. 373-381.

Hlastala MP, Woodson RD, *Bohr effect data for blood gas calculations*, J Appl Physiol. 1983 Sep; 55(3): p. 1002-1007.

Jensen FB, *Red blood cell pH, the Bohr effect, and other oxygenation-linked phenomena in blood O2 and CO2 transport*, Acta Physiol Scand. 2004 Nov; 182(3): p. 215-227.

Kister J, Marden MC, Bohn B, Poyart C, *Functional properties of hemoglobin in human red cells: II. Determination of the Bohr effect*, Respir Physiol. 1988 Sep; 73(3): p. 363-378.

Kobayashi H, Pelster B, Piiper J, Scheid P, *Significance of the Bohr effect for tissue oxygenation in a model with counter-current blood flow*, Respir Physiol. 1989 Jun; 76(3): p. 277-288.

Lapennas GN, *The magnitude of the Bohr coefficient: optimal for oxygen delivery*, Respir Physiol. 1983 Nov; 54(2): p.161-172.

Matthew JB, Hanania GI, Gurd FR, *Electrostatic effects in hemoglobin: Bohr effect and ionic strength dependence of individual groups*, Biochemistry. 1979 May 15; 18(10): p.1928-1936.

Meyer M, Holle JP, Scheid P, *Bohr effect induced by CO2 and fixed acid at various levels of O2 saturation in duck blood*, Pflugers Arch. 1978 Sep 29; 376(3): p. 237-240.

Monday LA, Tétreault L, *Hyperventilation and vertigo*, Laryngoscope 1980 Jun; 90(6 Pt 1): p.1003-1010.

Tyuma I, *The Bohr effect and the Haldane effect in human hemoglobin*, Jpn J Physiol. 1984; 34(2): p.205-216.

Winslow RM, Monge C, Winslow NJ, Gibson CG, Whittembury J, *Normal whole blood Bohr effect in Peruvian natives of high altitude*, Respir Physiol. 1985 Aug; 61(2): p. 197-208.

4.4 Less oxygen for cells

Summarizing the previous physiological laws, we can make the following conclusions:

1. **Hyperventilation or deep breathing cannot increase O2 content in the arterial blood to any significant degree (normal hemoglobin saturation is about 98%), but it reduces CO2 concentrations in all cells and the blood.**

2. **Hypocapnia (or CO2 deficiency)** (for more information, visit http://www.normalbreathing.com/d/hypocapnia.php) **leads to constriction of blood vessels and that reduces blood supply to vital organs of the human body.**

3. **Hypocapnia (or CO2 deficiency) also leads to suppressed Bohr effect that causes reduced O2 release in tissues and further reduction in delivery of O2 to cells.**

4. **Hence, the more one breathes, the less oxygen is provided for vital organs of the human body.**

The discussed effects of CO2-deficiency on blood flow and oxygen transport are summarized on the two graphs on the next two pages.

Normal gas exchanges

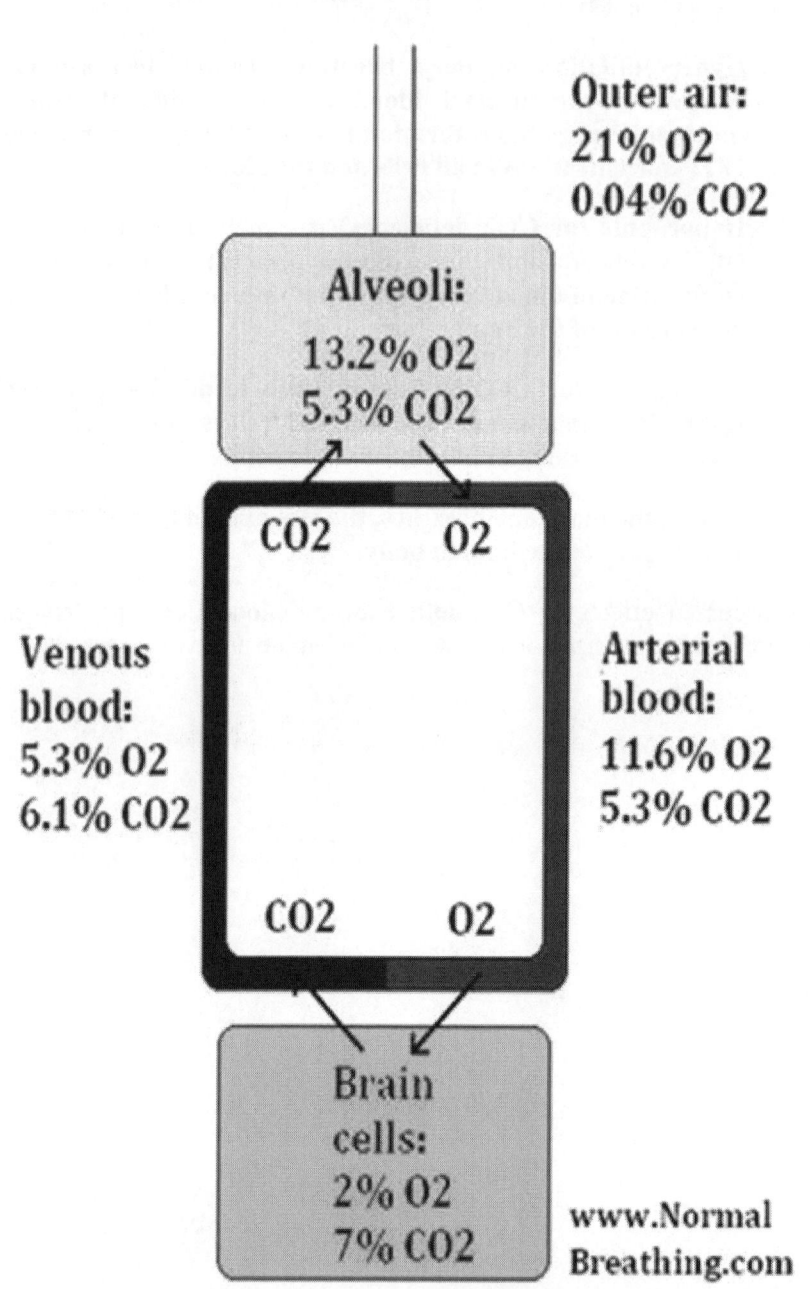

Outer air:
21% O2
0.04% CO2

Alveoli:
13.2% O2
5.3% CO2

CO2 O2

Venous blood:
5.3% O2
6.1% CO2

Arterial blood:
11.6% O2
5.3% CO2

CO2 O2

Brain cells:
2% O2
7% CO2

www.NormalBreathing.com

Effects of hyperventilation on circulation and normal gas exchange

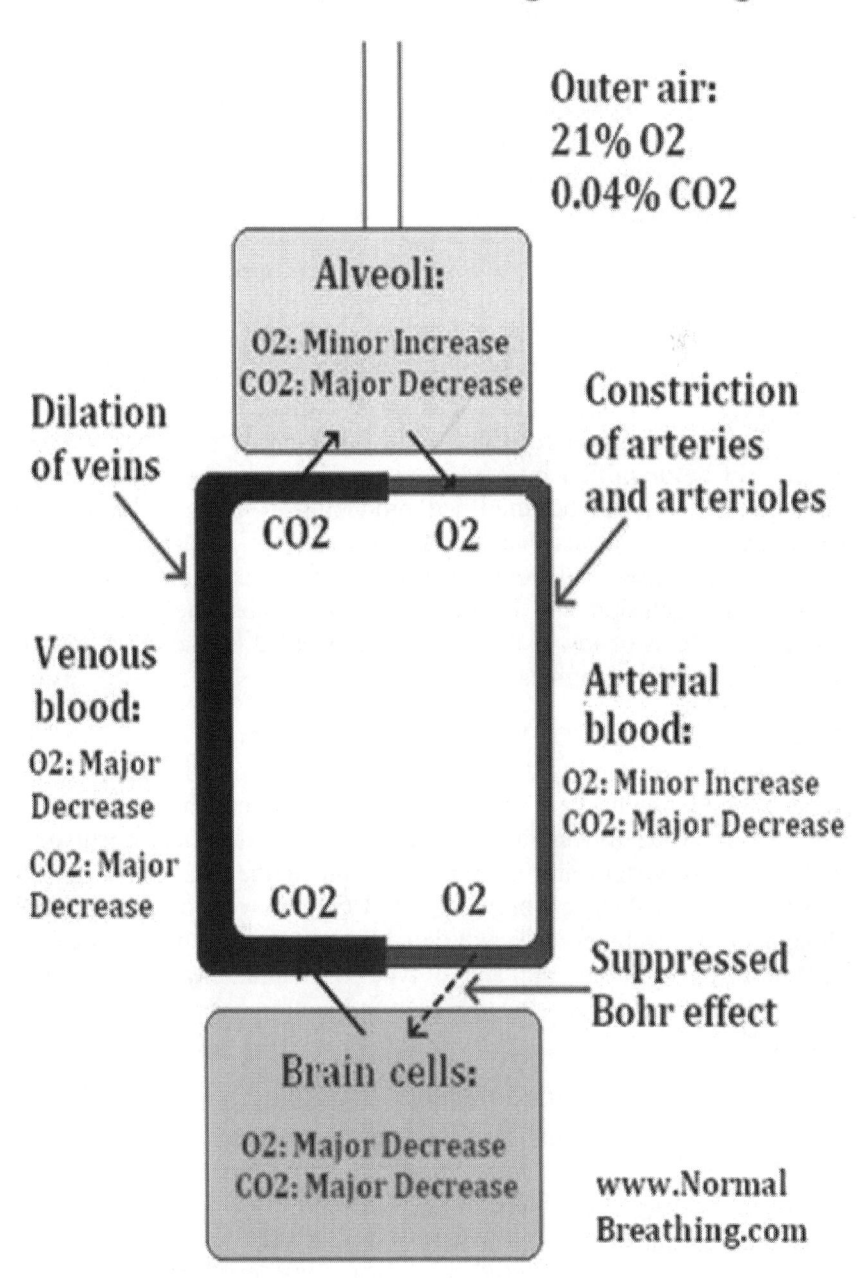

Outer air:
21% O2
0.04% CO2

Alveoli:
O2: Minor Increase
CO2: Major Decrease

Dilation of veins

Constriction of arteries and arterioles

CO2   O2

Venous blood:
O2: Major Decrease
CO2: Major Decrease

Arterial blood:
O2: Minor Increase
CO2: Major Decrease

CO2   O2

Suppressed Bohr effect

Brain cells:
O2: Major Decrease
CO2: Major Decrease

www.Normal Breathing.com

4.5 CO2 is crucial for mental health

"28. The breathing is calmed when the mind becomes steady and calm; ..." **Hatha Yoga Pradipika (15 century)**

Medical research proved an astonishing wisdom that is hidden in this short and simple phrase from yoga Sanskrit book written more than 500 years ago. Let us investigate the role of breathing in mental health and CO2 health effects (for more information, visit http://www.normalbreathing.com/CO2.php) on transmission of electrical signals between nerve cells.

In order to transmit only right or real nervous signals, the nerve cells have a certain threshold of excitability. The presence and value of this threshold prevent irrelevant or accidental signals from creating chaos in the whole nervous system. Indeed, imagine that there is no any threshold of excitability or it is too low. Then even a small accidental electrical signal will get a strong response from other nerve cells because the signals can be amplified by other nerve cells. As a result, such small accidental signals can be amplified producing a strong effect on the whole brain. This means that any strange idea or fantasy or a signal coming from senses and body organs may become a plan for future actions. Any delusion can be perceived as an absolutely real. Such destructive effects of low excitability are prevented by having a normal threshold that is, in mammals, is about 40 mV.

However, when brain CO2 becomes abnormally low, nerve cells suffer from abnormal excitability due to the lowered threshold. Therefore, CO2 is also called a tranquillizer or sedative of nervous cells that makes them calm. Normal CO2 concentrations create conditions for the normal work of the nervous system and normal reflection of the real world due to transmission of real signals only. Normal CO2 puts you in control of the whole nervous machinery to make right choices. Overbreathing naturally leads to low CO2 in the brain and all types of mental, psychological and psychiatric abnormalities since the ideas and fantasies appear as out from nowhere.

In the early 1950's, one of the world's leading physiological magazines, *Physiological Reviews*, published an extensive research article with the title "*Physiological effects of hyperventilation*". In this large article, Dr. Brown (Department of Physiology, University of Kansas Medical Center; USA) provided an analysis of nearly 300 professional physiological and medical studies. When considering the effects of carbon dioxide deficiency on the nerve cells, he wrote, *"Studies designed to determine the effects produced by hyperventilation on nerve and muscle have been consistent in their finding on increased irritability"* (Brown, 1953). Muscles and nerve cells become abnormally sensitive or irritated.

In 1965, *Journal of Physiology* (another leading physiological magazine) published the article titled "*Cortical CO2 tension and neuronal excitability*". It was shown that CO2 has a strong calming effect on excessive excitability of brain areas responsible for thinking (Krnjevic et al, 1965). Many other physiological studies confirmed this effect (Davis, Pascual & Rice, 1928; Necheles & Gerard, 1930; Lorente de No, 1947).

In 1988 physiologists from Duke University (Durham, the UK) suggested in their summary, *"The brain, by regulating breathing, controls its own excitability"* (Balestrino & Somjen, 1988).

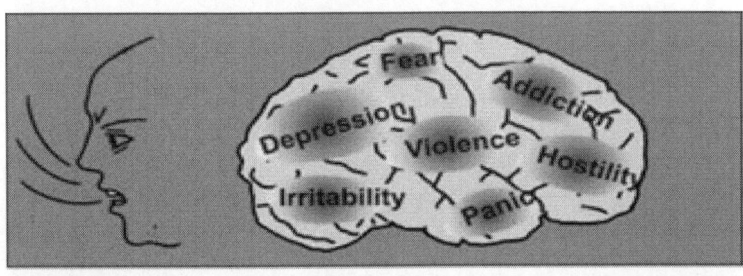

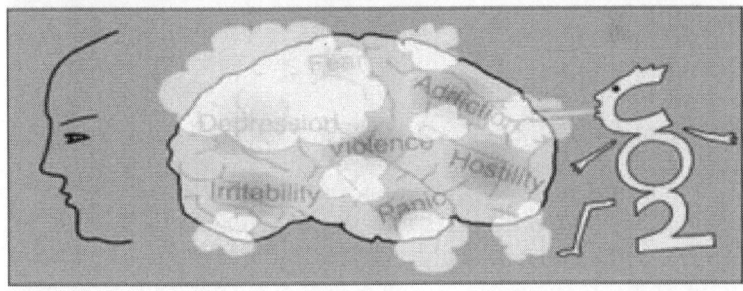

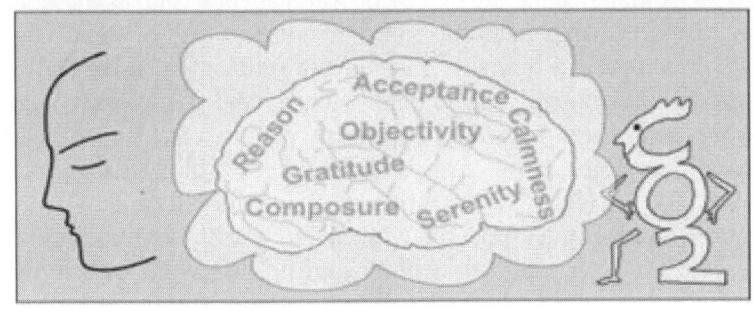

According to a recent study of Finnish scientists from the Laboratory of Neurology (University of Joensuu, Finland) **hyperventilation** *"leads to spontaneous and asynchronous firing of cortical neurons"* (Huttunen et. al, 1999). The study was published in the *Experimental Brain Research*. If you experience any of the problems related to anxiety, confusion, panic attacks, depression, insomnia or even addictions to coffee, sugar, alcohol, and many other substances, objects or activities (like computer games, gambling, and so forth), then you need to increase your brain CO_2 levels. Higher brain CO_2 will also raise your brain oxygenation leading to a dramatic improvement in your mental wellbeing.

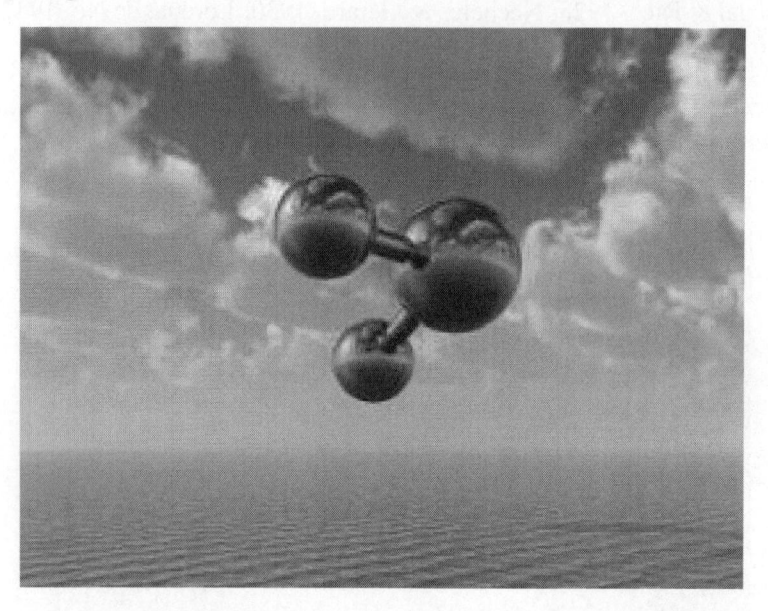

As a summary, we can conclude that low CO_2 prevents normal perception of reality and upsets stability of the nervous system. Instead of objective reflection and analysis of reality, in conditions of low CO_2, the brain starts to generate its own "spontaneous and asynchronous" ideas, projects, explanations, and interpretations of real events. Moreover, an excited brain cells can create problems that, in reality, do not exist. Hence, anxiety, fear, panic attacks, and many other negative emotions and states naturally appear in people who have breathing disorders (breathing problems or difficulties), while CO_2 is natural sedative (for more information, visit http://www.normalbreathing.com/CO2-stabilizer.php) and tranquilizer of nerve cells. It is crucial for stability and normal work of nerves and treatment-prevention of anxiety, stress, insomnia, phobias, and many other mental health problems.

There are dozens of other fascinating medical studies that back-up the wisdom of traditional yoga suggest calming the breath (see the yoga quote at the top of this Section). It is beyond the scope of this book to analyze all these medical articles that claimed presence of overbreathing and low CO_2 in people with various psychological and mental health problems. However, there are several titles in the second set of references that are provided below. Just titles alone testify the presence of the solid link between abnormal breathing and these health problems.

References

Balestrino M, Somjen GG, *Concentration of carbon dioxide, interstitial pH and synaptic transmission in hippocampal formation of the rat*, J Physiol 1988, 396: p. 247-266.

Brown EB, *Physiological effects of hyperventilation*, Physiol Reviews 1953 Oct, 33 (4): p. 445-471

Davis H, Pascual W, Rice LH (1928), *Quantitative studies of the nerve impulse*. Amer. J. Physiol. 86, 706-724.

Huttunen J, Tolvanen H, Heinonen E, Voipio J, Wikstrom H, Ilmoniemi RJ, Hari R, Kaila K, *Effects of voluntary hyperventilation on cortical sensory responses. Electroencephalographic and magnetoencephalographic studies*, Exp Brain Res 1999, 125(3): p. 248-254.

Krnjevic K, Randic M and Siesjo B, *Cortical CO_2 tension and neuronal excitability*, J of Physiol 1965, 176: p. 105-122.

Lorente DE (1947), *A study of nerve physiology*. Stud. Rockefeller Inst. med. Res. 131, pp. 148-193.

Necheles H & Gererd RW (1930), *The effect of carbon dioxide on nerve*, Amer. J. Physiol. 93, 318-336.

References
(Effects of hypocapnia on neurological symptoms and mental states)

Allen TE, Agus B. (1968) *Hyperventilation leading to hallucinations*. Am J Psychiatry 1968;125:632-7.

Bonn JA, Readhead CP, Timmons BH. *Enhanced adaptive behavioural response in agoraphobic patients pretreated with breathing retraining*. Lancet 1982;ii: 665-9.

Garssen B, Van Veenendaal W, Bloemink R. *Agoraphobia and the hyperventilation syndrome*. Behav Res Ther 1983;21:643-9.

Hibbert GA, *Hyperventilation as a cause of panic attacks*, Br Med J (Clin Res Ed) 1984 January 28; 288(6413): 263–264.

Ker WJ, Dalton JW, Gliebe PA. *Some physical phenomena associated with the anxiety states and their relation to hyperventilation*. Ann Intern Med 1937; 2: 962.

Ley R. *Agoraphobia, the panic attack and the hyperventilation syndrome*. Behav Res Ther 1985; 23: 79-81.

Lum LC. *Hyperventilation and anxiety states*. JR Soc Med 1981; 74: 1-4.

Magarian G. *Hyperventilation syndromes: infrequently recognized common expressions of anxiety and stress*. Medicine 1982; 61: 219-336.

Salkovskis PM, Warwick HMC, Clark DM, Wessells DJ. *A demonstration of acute hyperventilation during naturally occurring panic attacks*. Behav Res Ther 1986; 34: 91-4.

4.6 Other hypocapnia- and hypoxia-related effects

There are many other effects of low CO2 and O2 levels. For example, low CO2 leads to the following effects:

- irritable state of muscles (muscular tension) (Brown, 1953; Hudlicka, 1973)
- bronchoconstriction (for more information, visit http://www.normalbreathing.com/d/bronchoconstriction.php) (or reduced diameter of airways causing wheezing and sensations of breathlessness and suffocation) (for more information, visit (Buteyko, 1964; Herxheimer, 1946 and 1952; Sterling, 1968; Straub, 1998)
- abnormalities with ions in blood plasma and other bodily fluids (Carryer, 1947)
- innumerable abnormalities in chemical reactions involving synthesis of amino acids, lipids (fats), carbohydrates, hormones, messengers, cells of the immune system, etc.

If you suffer from asthma, or bronchitis, or cystic fibrosis, then CO2 is the key factor that will help you to prevent bronchospasm and increase body oxygenation.

As about too low levels of oxygen in body cells, the effects are also numerous. For example, low body oxygenation is the key factor in development and metastasis of cancer. Low O2 values in the heart tissue is the only factor that create angina pain. Numerous recent cutting-edge medical studies showed that cell hypoxia is the chief factor in development of diabetes and many other conditions.

Low O2 concentrations in cells prevent cells from recovery due to inflammation. In other words, cell hypoxia promotes chronic inflammation that is in the basis of numerous conditions, such as:

- arthritis and related conditions
- Alzheimer's disease
- bronchial asthma
- autoimmune diseases
- acne and related skin disorders
- allergic reactions
- atherosclerosis

(continues on next page)

(continued from previous page)

- chronic prostatitis
- Crohn's disease
- COPD
- dermatitis
- hepatitis
- hypersensitivities and allergic reactions
- insulin resistance (including diabetes)
- irritable bowel syndrome (IBS) of the intestinal tract
- inflammatory bowel diseases (IBD)
- lupus
- nephritis
- obesity
- cachexia
- gastrointestinal ischemia
- osteoarthritis
- pelvic inflammatory disease
- Parkinson's disease
- Sarcoidosis
- sleep apnea
- transplant rejection
- and ulcerative colitis.

Several other chronic diseases (including cancer, atherosclerosis, and ischemic heart disease) have their origins in chronic inflammatory processes.

If a yoga student wants to defeat these health problems, then improving body oxygenation by breathing correctly 24/7 is the smart way to go. Before analyzing these ways, we need to know how to measure body O2 content using a simple test.

References

Brown EB, *Physiological effects of hyperventilation*, Physiol Reviews 1953 Oct, 33 (4): p. 445-471.

Buteyko KP, A*n Instruction for VBN Therapy for Bronchial Asthma, Angina Pectoris, High Blood Pressure and Obliterating Endarteritis: Preprint.* - Novosibirsk, 1964.

Carryer HM, *Hyperventilation syndrome*, Med Clin North Amer 1947, 31: p. 845.

Herxheimer H, *Hyperventilation asthma*, Lancet 1946, 6385: p. 83-87.

Herxheimer H, *The late bronchial reaction in induced asthma*, Int Arch Allergy Appl Immunol 1952; 3: p. 323-328.

Hudlicka O, *Muscle blood flow*, 1973, Swets & Zeitlinger, Amsterdam.

Sterling GM, *The mechanism of bronchoconstriction due to hypocapnia in man,* Clin Sci 1968 Apr; 34(2): 277-285.

Straub NC, Section V, *The Respiratory System*, in *Physiology*, eds. RM Berne & MN Levy, 4-th edition, Mosby, St. Louis, 1998.

5. How to measure breathing and body oxygenation

5.1 Could we measure total body O2 using devices?

This graph below shows oxygen levels in one cross section of the human brain in two conditions: during normal breathing and after 1 minute of voluntary hyperventilation. The scale below provides exact numbers for each color.

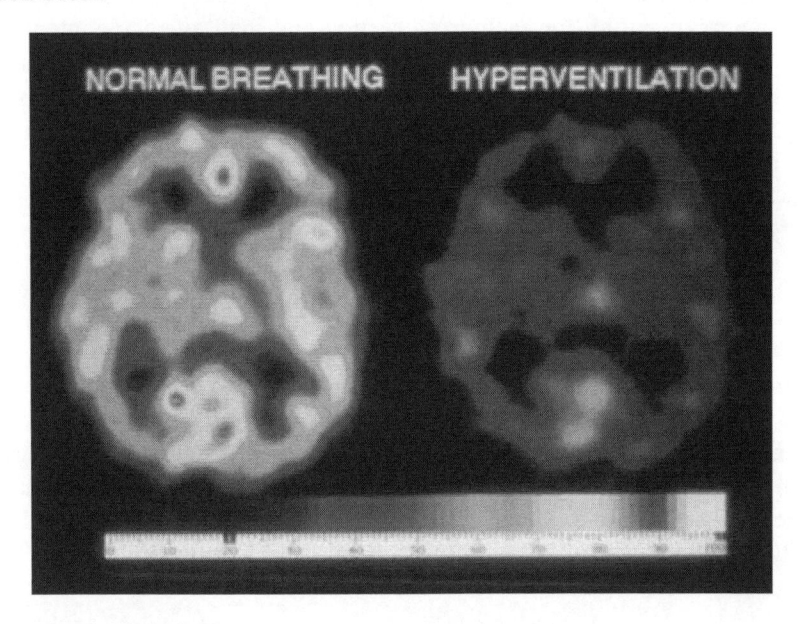

We can notice that, on both these images, oxygen distribution is very inhomogeneous. The most oxygenated area is located around the hypothalamus that is also known as the most ancient or primitive brain that is present even in simplest creatures, such as worms and bugs. The hypothalamus is responsible for primitive reflexes and bodily reactions, and it is generally the most active area of the brain. Since nerve activity requires more O2, the nature provided the hypothalamus with rich network of arteries to provide more blood and oxygen.

Depending on the situation and state of the human body, certain areas of the brain, similar to hypothalamus, can be more or less active requiring more or less oxygen, and this explains why this graph shows inhomogeneous oxygen distribution for normal breathing and hyperventilation that is present in more than 90% of modern people.

In addition, on a cell level, oxygen distribution among neighboring cells can also be very different. Those cells that are adjacent to capillaries can have high oxygen pressure (up to 4-5% or around 30-38 mm Hg). But more distant cells (some cells can be located as far away as 3-4 cells away from the nearest blood vessel) can have only 1% or about 7.6 mm Hg for oxygen partial pressure due to slow diffusion of oxygen through other cells that consume oxygen.

Therefore, it is very difficult to measure total brain O2 content. Even if we make thousands of similar PET scans for one brain, and then define average oxygenation for each cross section and then average content for the whole brain, there is a large factor related to this uneven cellular oxygen distribution. Even making one such image is a very expensive procedure that can cost hundreds of dollars. Obviously, making hundreds of similar PET scans is a very expensive procedure.

Total O2 content in the body

The situation with total body O2 content is even more complex. First of all, each organ and tissue has uneven O2 distribution. Besides, blood flow and O2 delivery to different organs are greatly influenced by the **autoregulation** effect that can change perfusion of certain organs up to 3-4 times. Autoregulation takes place due to various bodily processes, such as digestion, sleep, exercise, adaptation to temperature changes, emotions, local and global infections, local inflammation, and many others. Therefore, the total picture is very complex and, from the purely technical viewpoint, total body O2 content is exceptionally difficult and expensive to measure.

A simple DIY test to measure body O2 content

Leading Soviet physiologist Dr. Buteyko had devices to measure body O2 levels and knew about the effects described above when he worked as the Manager of the Laboratory of the Functional Diagnostic in Novosibirsk for first Soviet Spaceship Missions. Here is a photo of Dr. Buteyko with his staff members in his Laboratory in 1960's.

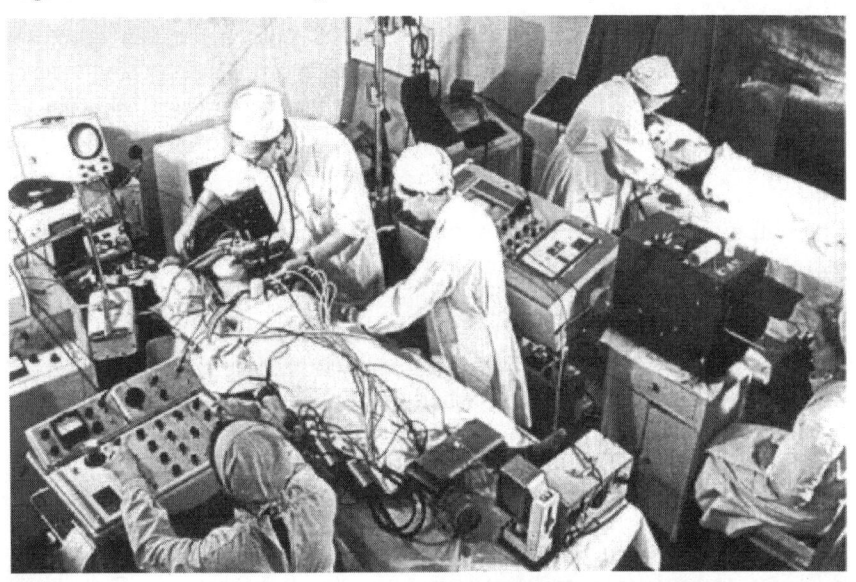

Yoga Benefits are in Breathing Less
Artour Rakhimov

He was surely interested in finding total body O2 content using his devices or other means. And he found a simple technique. After many years of research, he stated,

"Oxygen content in the organism can be found using a simple method: after exhalation, observe, how long the person can pause their breath without stress" Dr. K. P.Buteyko, "Dr. Buteyko lecture in the Moscow State University on 9 December 1969"

This statement is from a famous Buteyko's lecture in the Moscow State University. This special event was organized for the staff of the University. It was likely the classified nature of Buteyko's research during the 1960s (for first Soviet spaceship missions or Soviet Cosmos) and exclusiveness of his discoveries that predetermined the organization of this lecture (there was one more lecture, in 1972). Hence, it was definitely a very large and significant event for the scientific staff of the Moscow State University, the most famous and prestigious University of the USSR.

Later, this Lecture was republished in the very popular Soviet journal "Science and Life". Not many people are aware about the fact that the original title of this Lecture was "From incurable diseases to super-endurance of yogis" Furthermore, the Lecture quotes the term "yoga" more than 20 times or more often than all other health therapies combined and mentioned during this Lecture. Indeed, Dr. Buteyko studied yoga in details and practiced it himself for many decades later.

This Buteyko's observation about body O2 content makes common sense. When we hold our breath, we require more O2. But if you have certain O2 reserves, then we can comfortably tolerate breath holding ... until a certain point. Beyond this point in time, we suffer from stress and there is a growing desire to breathe.

The real picture is much more complex since CO2 is the main drive that increases ventilation (as during physical exercise). However, healthy people have higher CO2 and O2 at the same time, In addition, when one has more CO2 due to slower breathing, he or she is able to tolerate even higher CO2 values, while people with heavy breathing are hypersensitive to CO2 changes. And this is what the traditional yoga is all about: holding and restraining the breath to acquire very slow and light breathing at rest so that your body gets used to breathe less and have more O2 in cells.

5.2 Dr. Buteyko about yoga

Here are key quotes of Dr. Buteyko about yoga.

"There is one question not discussed here: what would happen with the organism, if breathing decreases below the norm? That is, when breathing changes from deep to shallow, and then from shallow to constantly shallow. Here we should not confuse full breathing of yogi with deep breathing.

Advocates of deep breathing confuse these two concepts and, in their defense, they say, "Yogi, for thousands of years, breathe deeply and we see that they are super-humans". Quite the contrary. Full breathing of yogi is shallow breathing in our understanding. It is done, first, very slowly, inhalations and exhalations as well; second, with maximum breath holds after inhalations and exhalations.

And finally one should not confuse the following concepts: we are speaking about breathing, which goes on day and night, about our basal breathing, foundation of life. Meanwhile, the system of yogi has separate breathing exercises. Therefore, it is practically unimportant for us how and what you do: feet upwards or downwards, through the right or left nostril, or by right or left side. We are interested in where you will arrive as a result of these exercises. If carbon dioxide increases, and breathing decreases, with each day, then this will ensure the transition of man into a super-endurance state.

Yoga Benefits are in Breathing Less
Artour Rakhimov

And if we record the lungs' ventilation and levels of carbon dioxide, it is clear that with such training lung ventilation is reduced, and carbon dioxide increases. Therefore, full breathing of yogi, according to its physiological effect, is analogous to our shallow breathing. This is the reason of its benefit. Now many people are interested in the systems of yogi. This, of course, is a surprisingly wise system of exercises.

I do not speak about any religions or superstitions, this is not part of the tasks of my lecture. But physiologically, yogi instinctively selected almost everything that decreases respiration: the majority of their postures (*asanas) lead to the decrease in respiration, and the respiratory gymnastics itself is called, in Indian, Pranayama. The literal translation means "slowing breath". Whatever the yogi did with their breathing, their final goal was to restrain [breathing], to harness it, to reach breathlessness and deathlessness. But those, who misinterpreted and badly understood it all, introduced this confusion that allegedly deep breathing is the breathing of yogi...

We declassified the major miracles of yogi. Their major miracles are in the reduction of respiration and accumulation of carbon dioxide. For thousands of years the yogi were looking for "prana", which is somewhere in food, air, etc. It turned out that carbon dioxide is prana. Here is the main source of life - carbon dioxide. If you accumulate it, you become a "superhuman"; if you lose it, you suffer....

There is no total one-sidedness: if we increase carbon dioxide above the norm (the middle norm), then an interesting phenomenon arises which I will explain later such as super-endurance [or super-resilience], a special stability of certain processes, a special stability of the nervous system, etc. Now we shall connect this with the secrets of yogi, which thus far have not been decoded. It turned out that we discovered the way to decipher super-resilience of yogi and their miracles.

All these miracles are based on the fact that yogis accumulate CO2, and all their secrets are connected with a reduction of breathing. Over 30 years ago [John] Haldane found that the organism regulates CO2 level with 0.1% accuracy (the threshold of CO2 regulation). Since this is the level of accuracy, CO2, obviously, is very important. Is oxygen regulated with the same precision? Only when oxygen decreases by more than 5%, the organism reacts to restore it.

Then we understood that by reducing breathing below the norm, our patients arrived at miracles. Here we realized . . . what it was all about!

It reminded of the yogi. What they strive for, it turns out, is achieved through reduction of breath and increase in carbon dioxide. This explains their miracles.

... Super-endurance of yogis is the effect of shallow breathing. This final result unites real yogis and our system, the scientific system of breathing. Yoga should be studied! There are many interesting physiological things there. This topic is raised by many scientists in Moscow, and I support them. We came across these phenomena accidentally, and if we focus on them, many interesting things can be discovered."

Extracts from **Dr. Buteyko Lecture in the Moscow State University** (1969) - http://www.normalbreathing.com/book-lecture.php.

5.3 How to measure body O2 (details)

Measurement of the CP (control pause)

Sit down and rest for 5-7 minutes. Completely relax all your muscles, including the breathing muscles. This relaxation produces natural spontaneous exhalation (breathing out). Pinch your nose at the end of this exhalation and count your CP (control pause or breath holding time) in seconds. Keep the nose pinched until you experience the first desire to breathe, so that, after you release the fingers, you can resume your usual breathing (in the same way as you were breathing just before you started to hold your breath). Do not extend breath holding too long. You should not gasp for air or open your mouth afterwards. The test should be easy and must not create any stress because it does not interfere with your breathing. Look at the diagram below: after the test you can comfortably breathe as before the test.

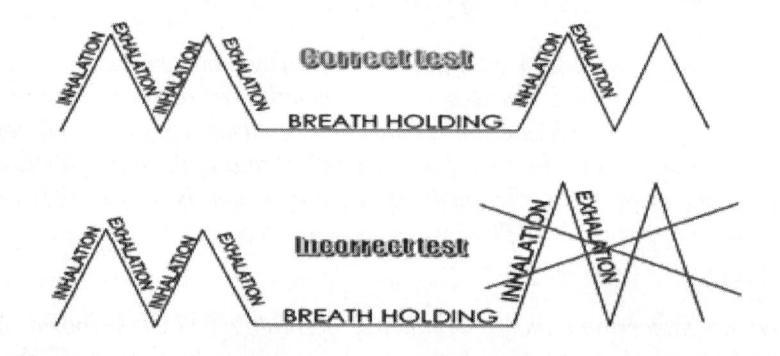

If you hold the breath for too long time (the incorrect test above), then your first inhale will be large, deep and noisy, as on the graph above.

I repeat again here since I have seen hundreds of people who try to get better numbers: **The test is done only until the first initial discomfort. You should have the same breathing pattern after the test as before the test: no gasping for air and no deep inhalations.**

If you get low numbers (e.g., about 15-20 seconds or even less), congratulations! Then you know what you need to improve: your most important health parameter or body O2 content.

Now you can easily define your health state at any moment of time. You can test various activities and how they influence body O2. Bear in mind though that physical exercise is an exception. It temporary reduces your current body O2, but increases next morning CP. We are going to discuss this effect later.

It was surely not accidental that breath holding is the breathing activity that is most commonly mentioned in ancient yoga books. You can easily find those traditional yoga books online for free and study them to be sure that breath holding is indeed the foundation of classical yoga. (Note that certain groups of people with panic attacks and hypertension should temporary avoid breath holding while practicing other activities that gradually improve their automatic breathing and increase O2 levels in cells. When they get up to about 25 s for body O2, then this test will be totally safe and stress-free for them.)

Since breathing patterns and body oxygenation change throughout the day, one's health parameters are usually worse during early morning hours. The MCP (morning control pause), according to Dr. Buteyko and his colleagues, is the main parameter that reflects personal health state. The MCP test is done as the first thing in the morning, while lying in bed, as soon as you open your eyes. My experience with hundreds of my students is the same: morning CP is the key parameters of one's health. It is important for future success, to write down your MCP every day. (The daily log is provided in below or can be downloaded from the website.) The next Section is devoted to the morning CP.

The CP is the simplest and most accurate test of personal physical health for more than 98% of people. This physiological fact has been confirmed by numerous studies and experiences of thousands of formerly-sick people who recovered their health using breathing retraining, especially the Buteyko method. Consider this graph with bars that summarize data from 9 independent medical publications. Each bar represents one physiological study with the title of the health condition and the number of patients (in brackets). The normal CP is about 40 seconds (the large bar on the left side). Shorter bars correspond to average numbers in people with chronic diseases.

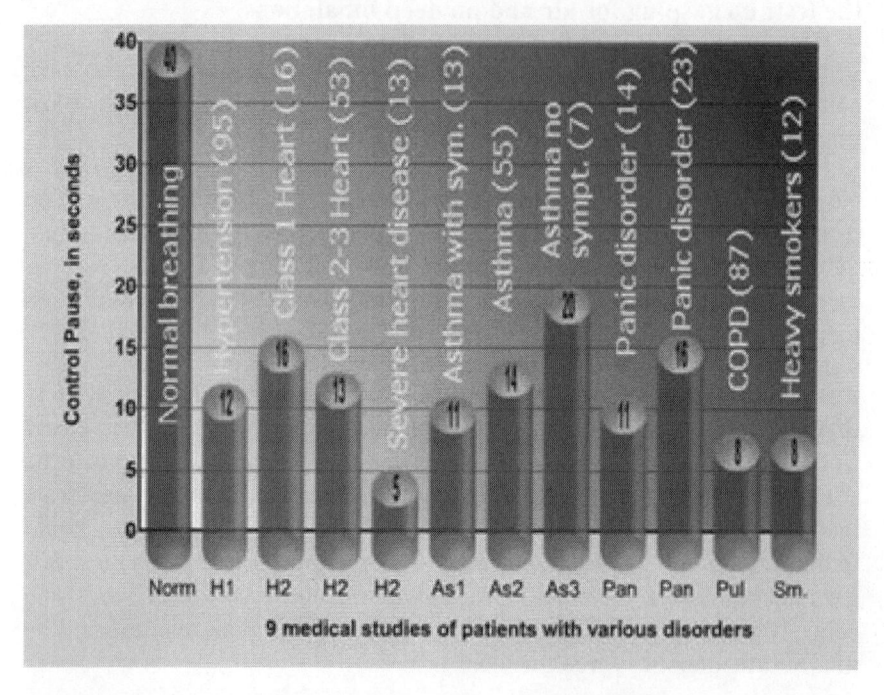

Note. For example, the second bar from the left represents a medical study in which it was found that 95 patients with hypertension had, on average, 12 seconds of oxygen in the body instead of normal 40 seconds. More details about the same studies are in these two Tables.

Condition	N. of subjects	Body O2	Reference
Hypertension	95	12 s	Ayman et al, 1939
Neurocirculatory asthenia	54	16 s	Friedman, 1945
Anxiety states	62	20 s	Mirsky et al, 1946
Class 1 heart patients	16	16 s	Kohn & Cutcher, 1970
Class 2-3 heart patients	53	13 s	Kohn & Cutcher, 1970
Pulmonary emphysema	3	8 s	Kohn & Cutcher, 1970
Functional heart disease	13	5 s	Kohn & Cutcher, 1970
Asymptomatic asthmatics	7	20 s	Davidson et al, 1974
Asthmatics with symptoms	13	11 s	Perez-Padilla et al, 1989
Panic attack	14	11 s	Zandbergen et al, 1992
Anxiety disorders	14	16 s	Zandbergen et al, 1992

Condition	N. of subjects	Body O2	Reference
Outpatients	25	17 s	Gay et al, 1994
Inpatients	25	10 s	Gay et al, 1994
COPD + congen heart failure	7	8 s	Gay et al, 1994
12 heavy smokers	12	8 s	Gay et al, 1994
Panic disorder	23	16 s	Asmudson & Stein, 1994
Obstructive sleep apnea	30	20 s	Taskar et al, 1995
Successful lung transplant	9	23 s	Flume et al, 1996
Successful heart transplant	8	28 s	Flume et al, 1996
Outpatients with COPD	87	8 s	Marks et al, 1997
Asthma	55	14 s	Nannini et al, 2007

We can also easily observe here that the oxygenation index correlates well with severity of the severity of the disease for asthma and heart patients. For example, functional heart disease corresponds to only about 5 miserable seconds of oxygen in the body, moderate heart disease (class 2 US classification) to about 10 second CP, and light forms of heart disease to about 15 seconds. Similarly, asthmatics who experience symptoms of asthma have about 10 seconds of oxygen. In between attacks (or in stable conditions), asthmatics usually have around 15 second for the body O2. If they get up to a 20 second CP, they do not experience chest tightness, wheezing, blocked nose and other pathological effects. Each and every student whom I taught also had these predicted values.

In both cases, asthma and heart disease, patients generally do not require any medication and do not experience any major symptoms when they get over 20 seconds 24/7. The same observation has been found for bronchitis, sinusitis, chronic fatigue, eczema, epilepsy and many other disorders.

Hence, the first goal for most patients, in order to get more stable health and reasonable well-being is to have over 20 second CP 24/7.

The CP test not only defines oxygenation of the human body, it also tells us about how heavy your breathing at rest right now is. If you have normal breathing, your CP should be around 40 seconds. If your CP is about 20 seconds, you breathe for 2 people. If your CP is 10 seconds, you breathe 4 times more than the medical norm.

Therefore, if you learn and practice some exercises, including pranayama and other yoga exercises, and do it correctly, you will gradually increase your body CO_2 content. Your CP will grow and your health will improve since your symptoms in relation to about 200 chronic diseases are controlled by your CP and breathing.

Clinical observations of over 100 Soviet and Russian physicians suggests that this CP test is simple and exceptionally valuable in order to define the current physiological state of the person, their symptoms and even requirements in medication. For a small portion of people (about 1% or less), this simple body oxygen test is not an accurate measure for their health due to very unusual circumstances, like surgical resection or accidental denervation of carotid nerve receptors, near death experience, and some other very rare cases.

References for the graph (in the same order)

Ayman D, Goldshine AD, *The breath-holding test. A simple standard stimulus of blood pressure*, Archives of Intern Medicine 1939, 63; p. 899-906.

Friedman M, S*tudies concerning the aetiology and pathogenesis of neurocirculatory asthenia III. The cardiovascular manifestations of neurocirculatory asthenia*, Am Heart J 1945; 30, 378-391.

Mirsky I A, Lipman E, Grinker R R, *Breath-holding time in anxiety state*, Federation proceedings 1946; 5: p.74.

Kohn RM & Cutcher B, *Breath-holding time in the screening for rehabilitation potential of cardiac patients*, Scand J Rehabil Med 1970; 2(2): p. 105-107.

Davidson JT, Whipp BJ, Wasserman K, Koyal SN, Lugliani R, *Role of the carotid bodies in breath-holding*, New England Journal of Medicine 1974 April 11; 290(15): p. 819-822.

Perez-Padilla R, Cervantes D, Chapela R, Selman M, *Rating of breathlessness at rest during acute asthma: correlation with spirometry and usefulness of breath-holding time*, Rev Invest Clin 1989 Jul-Sep; 41(3): p. 209-213.

Zandbergen J, Strahm M, Pols H, Griez EJ, *Breath-holding in panic disorder*, Compar Psychiatry 1992 Jan- Feb; 33(1): p. 47-51.

Gay SB, Sistrom C1L, Holder CA, Suratt PM, *Breath-holding capability of adults. Implications for spiral computed tomography, fast-acquisition magnetic resonance imaging, and angiography*, Invest Radiol 1994 Sep; 29(9): p. 848-851.

Asmundson GJ & Stein MB, *Triggering the false suffocation alarm in panic disorder patients by using a voluntary breath-holding procedure*, Am J Psychiatry 1994 Feb; 151(2): p. 264-266.

Taskar V, Clayton N, Atkins M, Shaheen Z, Stone P, Woodcock A, *Breath-holding time in normal subjects, snorers, and sleep apnea patients*, Chest 1995 Apr; 107(4): p. 959-962.

Marks B, Mitchell DG, Simelaro JP, *Breath-holding in healthy and pulmonary-compromised populations: effects of hyperventilation and oxygen inspiration*, J Magn Reson Imaging 1997 May-Jun; 7(3): p. 595-597.

Nannini LJ, Zaietta GA, Guerrera AJ, Varela JA, Fernandez AM, Flores DM, *Breath-holding test in subjects with near-fatal asthma. A new index for dyspnea perception*, Respiratory Medicine 2007, 101; p.246–253.

5.4 MCP (morning CP): your main health parameter

Physiological, medical and epidemiological studies have clearly shown that sick people are most likely to have acute exacerbations (due to heart attacks, strokes, asthma attacks, seizures, and others) during early morning hours. The same is true for chances of people with severe forms of heart disease, asthma, COPD, epilepsy, and many other conditions to die. Such tragic deaths due to diseases most likely to take place during early morning hours (4-7 am), when their breathing is the heaviest, body oxygenation is critically low, and the CP is about 5 seconds only or even less.

Now you can realize why more than 500 years ago, wise yoga masters wrote *"3. So long as the (breathing) air stays in the body, it is called life. Death consists inpassing out of the (breathing) air. It is, therefore, necessary torestrain the breath"* Hatha Yoga Pradipika (15 century). They noticed that many people die the hard way: i.e., with very heavy and fast breathing that makes O2 levels in the brain and heart critically low. My website has numerous studies showing that people with terminal (last stages of) cancer, HIV-AIDs, cystic fibrosis, and many other conditions have up to 30-40 breaths per minute for their respiratory frequency. Several studies measured CO2 content in the arterial blood and exhaled air in such critically ill people and found that it is nearly 2-3 times lower than the norm.

As about medical research related to Sleep Heavy Breathing Effect, you can visit the webpage "Morning Hyperventilation" (http://www.normalbreathing.com/index-MorningHV.php) or by watching my YouTube video-clip "How we breathe in the morning".

Most other people also experience the shortest CPs during early morning hours and feel worst in the morning after waking up. Possibly, this is the case with you too. Practical observations of Buteyko breathing doctors have confirmed that, indeed, in most people, up to 80% or more, their CPs significantly drops (up to 3-7 seconds or even more) during the night.

There are many causes that contribute to this Morning Hyperventilation effect. However, the very first aim for each person is to identify the presence and extent of this problem. How? Measure your CP immediately after waking up in the morning. As soon as you open your eyes, before getting out of the bed, do this DIY stress- free breath holding time test. Have a ticking or other clock or watch nearby to help you define your body O2 during last hours of sleep. The MCP (morning control pause), let me emphasize this once more, is the most important parameter of your physiological health.

5.4 Buteyko Table of Health Zones

Based on hundreds of medical studies, it is possible to suggest that the following effects take place with the progression of nearly any chronic disease:

- we breathe more air (minute ventilation increases)
- breathing frequency becomes higher
- breathing becomes deeper (tidal volume increases)
- CO2 content in blood decreases
- CP becomes shorter
- body oxygenation decreases
- heart rate increases.

These general effects are reflected in the **Buteyko Table of Health Zones** on the next page, that presents average parameters in people depending on their breathing.

Health state	Type of breathing	Degree	Pulse, beats/min	Breathing frequency/min	CO2 in alveoli, %	AP, s	CP, s	MP, s
Super-health	Shallow	5	48	3	7.5	16	180	210
		4	50	4	7.4	12	150	190
		3	52	5	7.3	9	120	170
		2	55	6	7.1	7	100	150
		1	57	7	6.8	5	80	120
Normal	Normal	-	60	8	6.5	4	60	90
Disease	Deep	-1	65	10	6.0	3	50	75
		-2	70	12	5.5	2	40	60
		-3	75	15	5.0	-	30	50
		-4	80	20	4.5	-	20	40
		-5	90	26	4.0	-	10	20
		-6	100	30	3.5	-	5	10

Table comments: Pulse – heart rate in 1 minute (all parameters are measured at rest); Rf – respiratory frequency in one minute (number of inhalations or exhalations in one minute); % CO2 - %CO2 in alveoli of the lungs (*or arterial blood if there is no mismatch); AP - the Automatic Pause or natural delay in breathing after exhalation (*during unconscious breathing); CP - the Control Pause, breath holding time after usual exhalation and until first distress; WP - Willful Pause, breath holding time from the first distress until the limit (after it, make frequent, but small inhalations while breathing through a slightly pinched nose); MP (the Maximum Pause, the sum of the CP and WP.

* **Note about heart rate:** Not all people have greatly increased heart rates, as is provided by this table, when parameters are at the bottom of the table or their CPs are low. Some categories of people with less than 20 second CP can have a resting pulse of around 60 - 70. However, increased heart rate for lower CPs is a feature of, for example, heart patients and patients with severe asthma. During the 1960's, when conducting his research, and later, Buteyko and his colleagues applied the Buteyko breathing retraining program mainly for heart and asthma patients, who were mostly hospitalized with frequent deficiencies in blood cortisol levels.

/ *This version is based on Buteyko KP, The method of volitional elimination of deep breathing [English translation of the Small Buteyko Manual], Voskresensk, 1994.*

Dr. Buteyko developed this table during 1960s, after analyzing hundreds of sick and healthy people in his respiratory laboratory, and presented it during his Lecture for the leading scientists at the Moscow State University in 1969. The Table reflects the health of his numerous hospitalized and severely sick patients, who started their journey for health at the very bottom of the table and climbed up, sometimes to the very top of the table. The top 5 zones were commonly known, among about 200 Soviet medical doctors, as the zones of super-endurance of yogi.

The middle row of the table corresponds to normal health. Below this row are 7 zones corresponding to disease. The borders for these zones are given by 7 rows (from normal down to "minus 6-th" degree). Five zones of yogi super-health are above the middle row. Let us start from the very bottom of this table and work up.

Terminally sick and critically ill patients during acute stages

The lowest row of this table corresponds to severely sick and terminally ill patients in critical conditions. When people are at the risk of dying, the table predicts over 100 beats per minute for their heart rate, over 30 breaths per minute for respiratory frequency, less than 3.5% CO_2 in the alveoli of the lungs. The CP (Control Pause or stress-free breath holding time after usual exhalation) is less than 5 seconds.

Terminally sick and critically ill patients in more stable conditions

The next row from the bottom corresponds to severely sick and terminally ill patients in stable conditions.

Typical heart rates of such people are above 90 beats per minute (sitting at rest). Respiratory rate (or breathing frequency) is above 26 breaths per minute at rest. A CO_2 concentration in alveoli of the lungs is no more than 4%. There is no automatic pause (period of no breathing after exhalation). The Control Pause is less than 10 seconds, while the Maximum Pause is less than 20 seconds. (Numerous medical studies confirmed that over 90% of patients with chronic diseases indeed die in conditions of severe hyperventilation, while their heart rate and respiratory frequency become much higher than the norms.

Quotes and exact numbers from such studies can be found on my website in relation to heart disease, asthma, cancer, and many other conditions.)

These patients usually require numerous types of medication to prevent their multiple symptoms and complaints. Due to heavy labored breathing, dyspnea, and low body oxygenation at rest, walking is hard and climbing stairs is often impossible. Most of the time is spent in bed, since even sitting requires effort.

Sleep is dreadful since breathing and symptoms get much worse after transition into a horizontal position.

Early morning hours (4-7 am) is the time when these patients are most likely to die from heart attack, stoke, asthma attack, or complications from cancer, diabetes, and many other pathologies.

Patients with moderate degree of their disease

The next row ("minus 4-th" degree of health) corresponds to patients whose life is not threatened at the moment, but their main concern are symptoms. People with mild asthma, heart disease, diabetes, initial stages of cancer, and many other chronic disorders are all in this zone. Taking medication is the normal feature for most of these people.

As we see from the table, heart rate for these patients varies from 80 to 90 beats per minute. Breathing frequency is between 20 and 26 breaths per minute (the medical norm is 12, while doctor Buteyko's norm is 8 breaths per minute at rest). CO_2 concentration in alveoli of the lungs is between 4.0 and 4.5%. The CP is between 10 and 20 seconds.

Physical exercise is very hard, since even fast walking results in very heavy breathing through the mouth, exhaustion, and worsening of symptoms. Complains about fatigue are normal. All these symptoms are often so debilitating that they interfere with normal life and the ability to work, analyze information, care about others, etc. Living in the chronic state of stress and being preoccupied with one's own miserable health are normal, while efficiency and performance in various areas (science, arts, sports, etc.) are compromised. Sitting in armchairs or soft couches is the most favorite posture.

Parameters of these people get worse during early morning hours with corresponding worsening of symptoms. Many sufferers get less than 10 seconds for the morning CP with all effects accompanying the last stage of the disease.

Most modern people

Most modern healthy people have between 20 and 30 second CP. Hence, they are going to be in the third row from the bottom ("minus 3-rd" degree of health). While there is no need for taking medication in this zone, numerous health pathologies are frequent. This relates to gastrointestinal disorders (gastritis, IBS, IBD, etc.), musculoskeletal problems (arthritis, osteoporosis, etc.), hormonal and metabolic problems (mild obesity, light diabetes), initial stages of cancer, and many others.

Standing for many hours is hard and they prefer to sit for most part of the day. Physical performance after meals is very poor since respiratory and cardiovascular parameters can shift to the lower zone. The level of energy and physical desire to work are low. The over-excited brain easily invents excuses for laziness. Morning parameters are much worse (less than a 20 second CP) with all effects that are present for this zone.

Normal health

As we continue to climb up the table, the next row corresponds to the norms. The row "minus 2" reflects international norms for breathing: breathing frequency of 12 breaths per minute; 5.5 % for CO2

concentrations in the alveoli of the lungs (about 41 mm Hg); 40 second CP and 70 beats per minute for heart rate. People with normal health naturally have a so called "automatic pause" or period of no breathing (total relaxation of all respiratory muscles after each exhalation) during their unconscious breathing. The duration of the automatic pause is about 2 seconds.

People with normal health are able to run with strictly nasal breathing, safely take a cold shower (if they follow certain other rules), have good quality sleep, and are reasonably able to function on the social level (family, community, workplace, etc.).

Buteyko norms

Dr. Buteyko suggested his own standards for health so that one can be free from about 200 chronic conditions. As we see in the table, healthy people should have a breathing frequency of no more than 8 breaths per minute at rest, more than 60 second CP, over 6.5% CO2, less than 60 beats per min for heart rate, and at least 4 seconds for the automatic pause.

At this stage people enjoy and even crave physical activity. They are full of energy (when they have a normal blood glucose level). Standing throughout the day is easy and natural. Sleep is less than 5 hours and early morning parameters are not worse than evening ones. All tissues of the body are histologically normal (or in accordance with medical books), while chronic disorders are impossible.

Stages that correspond to super-health

Buteyko also identified 5 stages that correspond to super-health or states related to "super-endurance of yogi" as they called them. Transition to the next row above the norm triggers certain biochemical processes and the appearance of lost abilities of the human body, including ability to digest wider varieties of fibers, painless childbirth, production of antibodies in saliva that prevent cavities and the formation of plague (no need to visit dentists 1-2 times every year), and some other effects. By the way, I was surprised to find out, may years ago, that yoga masters, according to yoga books, naturally required only 2 hours of sleep and did not need more sleep. When Dr. Buteyko and some of his MDs got up to 150-180 seconds CP, they also noticed the same effect: 2 hours of excellent refreshing sleep and no desire to sleep longer.

Buteyko generalized this table to a wide variety of conditions (heart disease, cancer, diabetes, asthma, and many others). He considered this table as an important discovery since he applied for a patent. His patent application is provided below.

RUSSIA (19)RU (11)99114075 (13)A (51) IPC7 **A61B5/00**

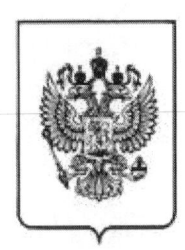

FEDERAL SERVICE FOR INTELLECTUAL PROPERTY,

Patents and Trademarks

(21), (22) Application:**99114075/14, 23.06.1999**

(43) Date of publication of application:**27.04.2001**

Address for correspondence: **121609, Moscow, Osennyi Boulevard, 11, (609 office), Company "CEP"**

(71) Applicant (s): **Veltistova Elena, Buteyko Konstantin Pavlovich (UA)**

(72) Author (s): **Veltistova Elena, Buteyko Konstantin Pavlovich (UA)**

(54)**METHOD OF ASSESSMENT OF HUMAN HEALTH**

(57) Abstract:

1. The method of assessing human health, including the definition of the parameters of functional systems and calculation of health indicators

based on the above parameters other than those that form the contingent of the surveyed people who determine the parameter information by measuring the breath holding time of the person after a usual exhalation before the first inhalation without following disturbances in breathing, and then determine and record the basic parameters of main functional systems, and each of them is compared with the informational parameter of the investigated person and obtain the parameter, which is a marker of major functional systems and / or indicator of human health, create a method to assess health through establishment of the scale, while comparing the actual values of each parameter of health survey with the normal value, and based on the received data, health groups can be formed.

2. The method, according to Paragraph 1, but is different in that the scale of health has five categories with a positive sign that characterize the health status of people with different levels of super- endurance and seven categories with a negative sign, which characterize the state of poor health and / or disease in humans with varying degrees of disease severity.

6. Yoga benefits in relation to chronic diseases

Dr. Buteyko was fascinated with wisdom of yoga. This is reflected in his Lecture that he delivered to leading scientists of the Moscow State University in 1969. While many hundred thousand people achieved normal or ideal health using the Buteyko method, Soviet and Russian Buteyko doctors knew that it is not what you do, but where you arrive due to your breathing retraining is the most important factor. Therefore, all his ideas are applicable to yoga benefits and health effects provided that one's automatic breathing pattern has been changed.

Here are chief clinical observations of Soviet and Russian doctors, as well as my own observations, that relate to health benefits (and yoga benefits) in relation to chronic diseases.

6.1 Respiratory diseases

- **Asthma**
    - An immediate decrease and, later, complete elimination of medication.
    - Increase in the CP is accompanied by normalization of immunity.
    - With the increased CP, allergic reactions become less severe and the number of allergens, which can provoke asthma attacks, decreases.
    - Improved physical endurance and improved quality of life.
    - Avoidance of triggers and high CPs (over 35 s 24/7) for 2-3 weeks lead to complete disappearance of allergies, disappearance of swelling and inflammation in airways, and normalization of lungs' tests.

- **Chronic bronchitis**
    - An immediate decrease and, later, elimination of the main symptoms of the disease (cough, dyspnea, heavy breathing, general tiredness, and fatigue).
    - Reduction in swelling and hyper-secretion from the mucosal surfaces of bronchi, and elimination of elements of bronchoconstriction.
    - Increase in the CP is accompanied by normalization of immunity.
    - Prevention of complications (e.g., pneumonia).
    - Significant improvements in the quality of life.
- **Acute respiratory diseases, including influenza and cold**
    - Reduction of recovery time from 5-7 days to 1-2 days.
    - Prevention of complications (e.g., sinusitis, laryngeal tracheitis, pharingitis, bronchitis, pneumonia, etc.).
    - Increase in the CP is accompanied by normalization of immunity.
    - Prevention of complications from chronic diseases, such as bronchial asthma, chronic obstructive bronchitis, hypertension, and myocardial ischemia.
- **Pneumonia**
    - An immediate decrease and, later, complete elimination of the main symptoms of the disease (cough and dyspnea) and symptoms of intoxication (general weakness and fatigue).
    - Increase in the CP is accompanied by normalization of immunity.
    - A decrease in swelling and hyper-secretion of mucus from the bronchi.
    - Significant reduction of the time of recovery.
- **Rhinitis, sinusitis**
  (frontal sinusitis, metopantritis, maxillary sinusitis)
    - Immediate complete or partial restoration of nasal breathing.
    - Decrease in doses of vasoconstrictive medications.
    - Prevention of appearance of pain and symptoms of intoxication.
    - Increase in the CP is accompanied by normalization of immunity and disappearance of inflammatory changes, decrease in swelling and hyper-secretion of mucus from the nasal passages, and decrease in frequency of acute episodes of the disease.
    - Surgical interventions become unnecessary.

- **Emphysema**
    - Immediate prevention of progression of the disease, improvement in arterial blood oxygenation tests, and reduction in medication (e.g., cortisol, beta-antagonists, etc.).
    - With the increased CP, gradual reduction in production of mucus, if it was present, ability to walk faster with nasal breathing, and improved ability to walk upstairs.
    - Use of oxygen 24/7 or lung transplantation becomes unnecessary.
    - Years of high CP (about 35 s or more) 24/7 result in gradual regeneration of alveoli and complete restoration of the lungs with normal X-ray results.
    - Significant improvements in the quality of life.

6.2 Cardiovascular diseases

- **Hypertension (primary)**
    - Immediate elimination of symptoms connected with elevated blood pressure: headache, dizziness, heart palpitations, pain near the heart, shivering, general fatigue, etc.
    - In cases of 1st or 2nd class hypertension, increase in the CP is accompanied by normalization of blood pressure, gradual elimination or significant reduction in doses of medications that reduce blood pressure (or transition from multi-medication to mono-therapy). In cases of 3rd class hypertension, it is possible to significantly reduce medications or make transition to mono-therapy.
    - When the CP is 20-30 s or more, the symptoms are absent and no medication is required. This usually takes less than 1-2 months of practice.
    - Natural weight normalization.
    - Prevention of insulin resistance, diabetes mellitus, hyperlipidemia, and hypertrophy of the left ventricle.
    - Prevention of injuries in targeted organs during 1st stage of the disease (myocardial infraction, stroke, angiogenesis of retina, nephropathy, etc.).

- **Ischemic heart disease**
    - Immediate elimination of symptoms of stenocardia attacks (angina pectoris) and prevention of their appearance (or decrease in angina-like pains).

- Increase in the CP is accompanied by transfer from the current functional class of the disease to a less severe one.
- Increase in the CP is accompanied by reduction and elimination of medication (to reduce angina-like pain)
- Significant improvements in the quality of life.

- **Heart failure**
  - Increase in the CP is accompanied by reduction of the symptoms of chronic cardiac insufficiency (edema of lower extremities, panting, heart palpitations, heartache, general fatigue, tiredness, etc.)
  - Increase in the CP is accompanied by decrease in the doses of medications and their number, natural reduction in triglycerides and cholesterol.
  - Significant improvements in the quality of life.

- **Arrhythmia**
  - Immediate elimination of heart palpitations and various accompanying symptoms: unpleasant feelings and pains near the heart, feelings of breathlessness and panting, chill and sweating, general fatigue, etc.
  - In cases of chronic forms of tachycardia, increase in the CP is accompanied by steady reduction in the heart rate, recovery of coronary circulation, and perfusion of injured parts of myocardium. That prevents reappearance of paroxysms of pulsating arrhythmia, ventricular tachycardia, etc.
  - Significant improvements in the quality of life.

- **Varicose veins**
  - Immediate decrease and, later, elimination of unpleasant symptoms: heaviness and leg cramps, puffiness around the feet, and weakness and fatigue of the lower extremities.
  - Increase in the CP is accompanied by decrease in the extent of the capillary bed and enlarged veins.
  - Prevention of possible complications due to chronic venous insufficiency: trophic ulcers, thromboembolism, and varicose eczema.
  - Significant improvements in the quality of life.

- **Dystonia**
  - Immediate decrease and, later, complete normalization of blood pressure and eliminate various symptoms (sweating, heart

palpitations, feelings of inner shivering and obstructed throat, etc.).
- Increase in the CP is accompanied by normalization of emotional life, restoration of sleep, disappearance of pains and aches in various body parts.
- Significant improvements in the quality of life.

6.3 Hormonal conditions

- **Diabetes mellitus**
    - Immediate decrease in insulin dosage twofold, use of insulin of short duration.
    - Increase in the CP is accompanied by decreased requirements in insulin and, at 35-40 s CP its complete elimination.
    - Prevention of complications.
    - High CP values (over 35 s) 24/7 lead to complete clinical remission (cure). The time of recovery is usually about 1/10 of the disease time (use of insulin).
    - Normalization of the emotional life of the students and significant improvement in the quality of life.

- **Hypothyroidism**
    - Immediate intensification of metabolism, energy level, and reduction in the thyroidal hormone dose
    - Increase in the CP is accompanied by increased energy, disappearance of possible feeling cold (e.g., cold extremities) and other negative symptoms.
    - High CP values (over 35 s) 24/7 lead to complete clinical remission and no need for medication.
    - Prevention of complications.
    - Significant improvements in the quality of life.

- **Obesity**
    - Immediate intensification of metabolism and changes in dietary preferences in the direction of "healthier" choices (eating less with better energy).
    - Increase in the CP is accompanied by redistribution of fat with its subsequent metabolism and increase in the muscular mass due to the catabolic effect.
    - With the increased CP, the ability and desire to exercise is gradually restored. Moreover, use of physical exercise leads to dramatic acceleration of the recovery rate.

- Prevention of complications.
- Significant improvements in the quality of life.

6.4 Gastrointestinal problems

- **Chronic gastritis**
  - Immediate decrease and, later, complete elimination of pain and symptoms due to dyspeptic effects (heartburn, regurgitation, nausea, etc.).
  - Increase in the CP is accompanied by normalization of colonic tone, phasic contractility of the GI tract, perfusion, metabolic processes in the mucosal surface of the esophagus and stomach causing accelerated healing of erosions and ulcers, together with regeneration of the mucosal surface of the stomach.
  - When the student achieved 35 s morning CP and maintained this level for more than 2 weeks, normalization of the immune profile leads to eradication of Helicobacter Pylori.
  - Prevention of complications due to chronic gastritis, and complete clinical remission for many years (cure).
  - Significant improvements in the quality of life.

- **Chronic non-ulcerative colitis**
  - Immediate decrease and, later, complete elimination of pain and symptoms due to dyspeptic effects (bloating and rumbling in the belly, regurgitation, nausea, inconsistencies in bowel habits, etc.).
  - Increase in the CP is accompanied by normalization of colonic tone, phasic contractility of the GI tract, perfusion, and metabolic processes in the mucosal surface leading to its regeneration.
  - When the student achieved 40 s CP or more and maintained this level for more than 2 weeks, normalization of the immune profile leads to normalization of the GI flora with elimination of pathogenic bacteria and inflammation in the lining of the large intestine.
  - Prevention of complications.
  - Complete clinical remission for many years (cure).
  - Significant improvements in the quality of life.

- **Chronic pancreatitis**
  - Immediate decrease and, later, complete elimination of pain and symptoms due to dyspeptic effects (bloating and rumbling in the

belly, regurgitation, nausea, vomiting, alternating bowel habits, etc.).
- Increase in the CP is accompanied by normalized colonic tone, phasic contractility of the GI tract and recovered internal secretion.
- Prevention of complications (diabetes mellitus, pancreonecrosis, secondary diseases of the biliary tract, etc.).
- Complete clinical remission for many years (cure).
- Significant improvements in the quality of life.

- **Chronic cholecystitis**
  - Immediate decrease and, later, complete elimination of pain and symptoms due to dyspeptic effects (bloating and rumbling in the belly, regurgitation, nausea, vomiting, alternating bowel habits, etc.)
  - Increase in the CP is accompanied by normalization of colonic tone, phasic
  - contractility of the GI tract, perfusion, metabolism in the lining of the intestine, tone of the bile-conducting organs and elimination of inflammatory processes in the bile-conducting system.
  - When the student achieved 35 s morning CP and maintained this level for more than 2 weeks, normalization of the immune profile leads to normalization of the GI flora, disappearance of pathogenic bacteria and elimination of inflammation in the biliary tract.
  - Prevention of complications. Inhibition of formation of stones in the gallbladder.
  - Complete clinical remission for many years (cure).
  - Normalization of the emotional life of the students and significant improvement in the quality of life.

- **Gastro-esophageal reflux (GERD)**
  - Immediate decrease and, later, complete elimination of pain and symptoms due to dyspeptic effects (heartburn and regurgitation).
  - Increase in the CP is accompanied by improved perfusion and normalization of the metabolic processes in the mucosal surface of the esophagus and stomach, with accelerated healing of erosions and ulcers.
  - When the student achieved 35 s morning CP and maintained this level for more than 2 weeks, normalization of the immune profile leads to normalization of the GI flora, disappearance of

pathogenic bacteria and elimination of inflammation in the biliary tract.
- Prevention of recurring appearances of erosions and ulcers.
- Normalization of the emotional life and significant improvement in the quality of life.

6.5 Diseases of kidneys and urinary tract

- **Chronic pyelonephritis**
    - Quick elimination of the symptoms (pain and unpleasant sensations during urination, frequent urination, etc.).
    - Decrease in the duration of antibacterial therapy and the achievement of positive results using mono-therapy (e.g., use of a single antibiotic medication).
    - In case of chronic states of the disease, the CP growth gradually increases parameters of the immunity.
    - Prevention of development of acute complications due to chronic pyelonephritis, and, in future, complete recovery.
    - Prevention of more severe forms of pyelonephritis (obstructive urinary pathologies, i.e., urinary stones, polycystic kidney disease, urinary tract reflux, benign prostatic hyperplasia, etc.) and structural changes in the kidneys and urinary tract, as a result of diabetes mellitus, neutropenia, kidney disease, polyarthritis, and other severe conditions.
    - Regression of the obstructive effects, pH normalization, prevention of appearance of new stones, and dissolution of old stones and their elimination.
    - Significant improvements in the quality of life.

- **Kidney and urinary stones**
    - Quick elimination of the symptoms (pain, unpleasant sensations due to presence of stones in the urinary tract).
    - With the increased CP, gradual normalization of the urinary pH, ability to hold more urine without any symptoms, and disappearance of symptoms of the disease
    - Prevention of shock wave therapy, surgery, and medication. Prevention of complications.
    - Significant improvements in the quality of life.

6.6 Diseases of the musculoskeletal system

- **Osteochondrosis**
    - Elimination of the symptoms (pain and unpleasant sensations due to bony necrosis).
    - With the increased CP, gradual normalization of restorative processes in the affected areas and bone re-growth.
    - High CPs (over 35 s) for some weeks result in healing of the bone in a relatively normal shape and absence of any symptoms.
    - Prevention of surgery, as in case of Legg-Calvé-Perthes disease, and the need for joint replacement.
    - Prevention of complications (e.g., arthritis).
    - Significant improvements in the quality of life.

- **Polyarthritis**
    - Immediate reduction or elimination of pain.
    - With the increased CP, gradual reduction in joint swelling, and their stiffness and restrictions of movements.
    - When the student achieved 35 s morning CP and maintained this level for some weeks, normalization of the regenerative processes in the affected areas leads to elimination of degenerative processes, inflammation, and joint damage and complete disappearance of symptoms.
    - Prevention of surgery and the need for joint replacement.
    - Prevention of complications.
    - Normalization of the emotional life of the students and significant improvements in the quality of life.

- **Chronically poor healing of bone fractures**
    - Immediate reduction or elimination of pain.
    - With the increased CP, gradual reduction in possible swelling, stiffness, and restrictions of movements.
    - When the student achieved 35 s morning CP and maintained this level for some weeks, normalization of the regenerative processes in the affected areas leads to elimination of degenerative processes, inflammation, and healing of the fracture and complete disappearance of symptoms.
    - Prevention of surgery and the need for joint replacement. Prevention of complications.
    - Significant improvements in the quality of life.

6.7 Skin diseases

- **Eczema**
  - Immediate decrease, and with higher CP, total elimination of skin itching.
  - Normalization of psychological and emotional states of the student.
  - Increase in the CP and its maintenance within 30-40 s range are accompanied by gradual decrease in the area of skin rash with its subsequent complete disappearance.
  - Significant improvements in the quality of life.

  - **● Psoriasis**
  - Immediate decrease, and with higher CP, total elimination of skin itching.
  - Normalization of psychological and emotional states of the student.
  - Increase in the CP and its maintenance within 30-40 s range are accompanied by gradual decrease in the area of skin rash with its subsequent complete disappearance.
  - Prevention of complications (arthropathy, psoriasis erythrodermia, skin infections, amyloidosis, etc.).
  - Improvement of the general state of the students (stabilization of the respiratory symptoms of the allergy and the dynamic of the accompanying chronic diseases, i.e. diseases of the GI tract, chronic infections, etc.).
  - Significant improvements in the quality of life.

- **Neurodermitis**
  - Immediate decrease, and with higher CP, total elimination of skin itching.
  - Normalization of psychological and emotional states of the student.
  Increase in the CP and its maintenance within 30-40 s range are accompanied by gradual decrease in the area of skin rash with its subsequent complete disappearance.
  - Restoration of the sleep (in cases of its abnormalities).
  - Improvement of the general state of the students (stabilization of the symptoms of the allergy, such as rhinoconjunctivitis, symptoms of bronchial obstruction, etc.).
  - Significant improvements in the quality of life.

6.8 Allergies and Immunodeficiency

- **For allergic rhinitis and nasal polyps**
    - Immediate restoration of nasal breathing, decrease in nasal discharges, decrease in the dosages and frequency of application of vasoconstrictive medication.
    - The growth of the CP is accompanied by stable remission with complete elimination of swelling, medication and full restoration of nasal breathing.
    - Prevention of surgery.
    - Normalization of the emotional life of the students and significant improvement in the quality of life.
    - **● Allergic conjunctivitis**
    - Immediate reduction of symptoms (e.g., itching) and decrease in the amount of medication.
    - The growth of the CP is accompanied by complete elimination of skin itching, decrease the area covered with rash, and decrease the duration of use of medication.
    - Normalization of the emotional life of the students and significant improvement in the quality of life.
    - **● States of immunodeficiency (secondary)**
    - Immediate elimination of clinical symptoms of secondary immunodeficiency, such as frequent infective and inflammatory processes in the lungs, bronchi, nasal passages, urinary system, GI tract, eyes, skin, and soft tissues.
    - Further CP growth prevents development of similar complications.
    Significant improvements in the quality of life.
    - Transition of children and adults from the "frequently sick" category into the "practically healthy" one.

7. Other yoga benefits due normalization of breathing

Although the effects of chronic hyperventilation are variable and individual, there are certain changes that are experienced by most people who either normalized their breathing or have made certain progress in this direction. These changes are summarized below.

7.1 Physiological and neurological changes

- These changes are based on the more stable autonomic nervous system, with a tendency toward parasympathetic dominance (rather than the usual stress-induced sympathetic dominance). That usually includes the following changes:
- respiratory efficiency increases (respiratory rate decreases, respiratory amplitude and tidal volume decreases (for the CPs up to 1-2 min), breathing smoothness increases, vital capacity increases, FEV increases)
- cardiovascular efficiency increases (pulse rate and blood pressure decrease)
- electrical skin resistance decreases ((less sweating, more relaxation)
- EEG changes: alpha waves increase (theta, delta, and beta waves also increase during various stages of the breathing exercises)
- EMG activity decreases
- gastrointestinal function normalizes ((gut flora improves, intestinal tone normalizes, stool consistency improves, bowel movements become easier and more regular, constipation disappears)
- skin gets stronger, shining, more resilient and elastic (sebaceous glands produce more oil); skin rashes, skin sagging, easy skin bruising, skin dryness and noxious sweat odor disappear; wound healing time is decreased

- skin flora, skin respiration, skin sensations, and skin excretory functions improve
- wound-healing time and accompanied inflammation around wounds decrease
- water balance and kidney function improve (less water is required for proper hydration, urinary frequency decreases and urinary volume increases, puffiness and excessive water retention disappears)
- various endocrine functions normalize (energy level increases, weight normalizes, appetite improves)
- sleeping quality improves (less time is required for falling asleep; sleeping time is decreased; more time is spent in deep, dreamless sleep; the number of awakenings is smaller (down to 0 when the CP is above 60 s); less or no discomfort or pain is experienced; the number of body's movements and changing positions during the sleep is decreased (down to 0))
- musculoskeletal and joint flexibility increases posture improves
- strength and resiliency increase endurance increases
- immunity increases
- pain threshold increases.

7.2 General psychological and social changes

Psychological changes are manifested in more efficient work of the nervous system and permanent changes in personal attitudes towards surrounding environment, self, and other people. These changes are possible due to increased blood supply to the brain (section 1.4) and increased threshold of neuronal excitability (also section 1.4). The person has an increased ability to remain calm under stressful conditions. Among these are the following changes:

- anxiety and depression decrease, mood swings disappear
- self-acceptance and self-actualization increase
- cognitive function and perception improve
- attention, concentration, memory (both, short and long-term), learning efficiency, and various logical abilities improve
- more objective perceptions of the outside world, other people, own place in this world, and own abilities and limitations are possible
- hostility decreases

- tolerance and social adjustment increases
- addictions, cravings, and unhealthy attachments disappear
- the desire to find the truth and essence of objects, processes and activities increases.

7.3 Biochemical effects

Normalization of various biochemical processes is revealed in the following changes (these are confirmed by blood analysis):
- blood glucose and insulin levels decrease, insulin sensitivity increases
  plasma sodium decreases
- total cholesterol decreases (triglycerides decrease, HDL cholesterol increases, LDL cholesterol decreases, VLDL cholesterol decreases, cholinesterase increases)
- thyroxin level and ATPase increase
- hematocrit and hemoglobin level increase
- lymphocyte count increases, total white blood cell count decreases
- total serum protein increases.

7.4 Technical skills

Changes in technical skills are possible due to better communication between the nervous system and muscles. Various technical and psychomotor functions improve, including:
- dexterity and fine motor skills
- grip strength
- eye-hand coordination
- reaction time and choice reaction time
- steadiness and balance
- execution of complicated movements.

7.5 Changes in physical and general sport skills

Psychology-related and physiology-related changes are also manifested in improvements in various physical and sport skills. They are based on domination of subcortical regions of the brain and domination of the parasympathetic part of the autonomic nervous system. These changes are in comparison with previous states (corresponding to chronic hyperventilation) during similar physical exercise. It can be noticed and often measured that now the person has:

- more accurate and goal-oriented movements ((in the past, the movements during the periods of depression were too slow, while during excitements and bursts of activities were too fast and imprecise)
- normalization of muscle tone
- lower risk of injuring muscles and ligaments
- lower energy spending (efforts are minimum, irrelevant muscles and the rest of the body are more relaxed, activity of opposing muscle groups is more balanced)
- increased maximum oxygen uptake
- increased maximum tolerated lactate level
- non-competitive, goal-oriented, more detached and objective attitude.

7.6 Lifestyle changes as yoga benefits

Meanwhile, there are truly amazing changes that took place with every person who gets high CPs. This Table shows some of these changes.

Lifestyle factor:	Body O2 < 30 s	Body O2 > 50 s
Energy level	Medium, low, or very low	High
Desire to exercise	Not strong, but possible	Craving and joy of exercise
Intensive exercise with nose breathing	Hard or impossible	Easy and effortless
Typical mind states	Confusion, anxiety, panic, depression	Focus, concentration, clarity
Craving for coffee, sugar and junk foods	Present	Absent
Addictions to smoking, alcohol, and drugs	Possible	Absent
Desire to eat raw foods	Weak and rare	Very common and natural
Correct posture	Rare and requires efforts	Natural and automatic
Sleep	Often of poor quality; > 7 hours	Excellent quality; < 5 hours naturally

Apart from these changes, there are many others such as painless childbirth, ability to digest much wider varieties of foods, natural reduction in sleep (down to 2 hours at very high CPs), and some others that were and are normal among real yoga masters.

8. Key practical steps in breathing retraining to get yoga benefits

How can a yoga student apply this key yoga secret in real life? Of course, the purpose is to increase body O2 and achieve real health that was common among yoga masters for centuries. Practically, when I teach breathing retraining, there are several intermediate goals in health improvement.

Level 1. No exacerbations of chronic diseases

Severely sick people need to learn simple breathing exercises to stop their exacerbations. Since they commonly have about 10 s CP, this is only a temporary relief that does not provide good health but helps to reduce medication and have less serious symptoms.

Level 2. Stable health

Most sick people can eliminate their main symptoms and medication if they get over 20 s CP 24/7. On the next page is an infograph detailing the main requirements for getting higher CP that I use for breathing retraining.

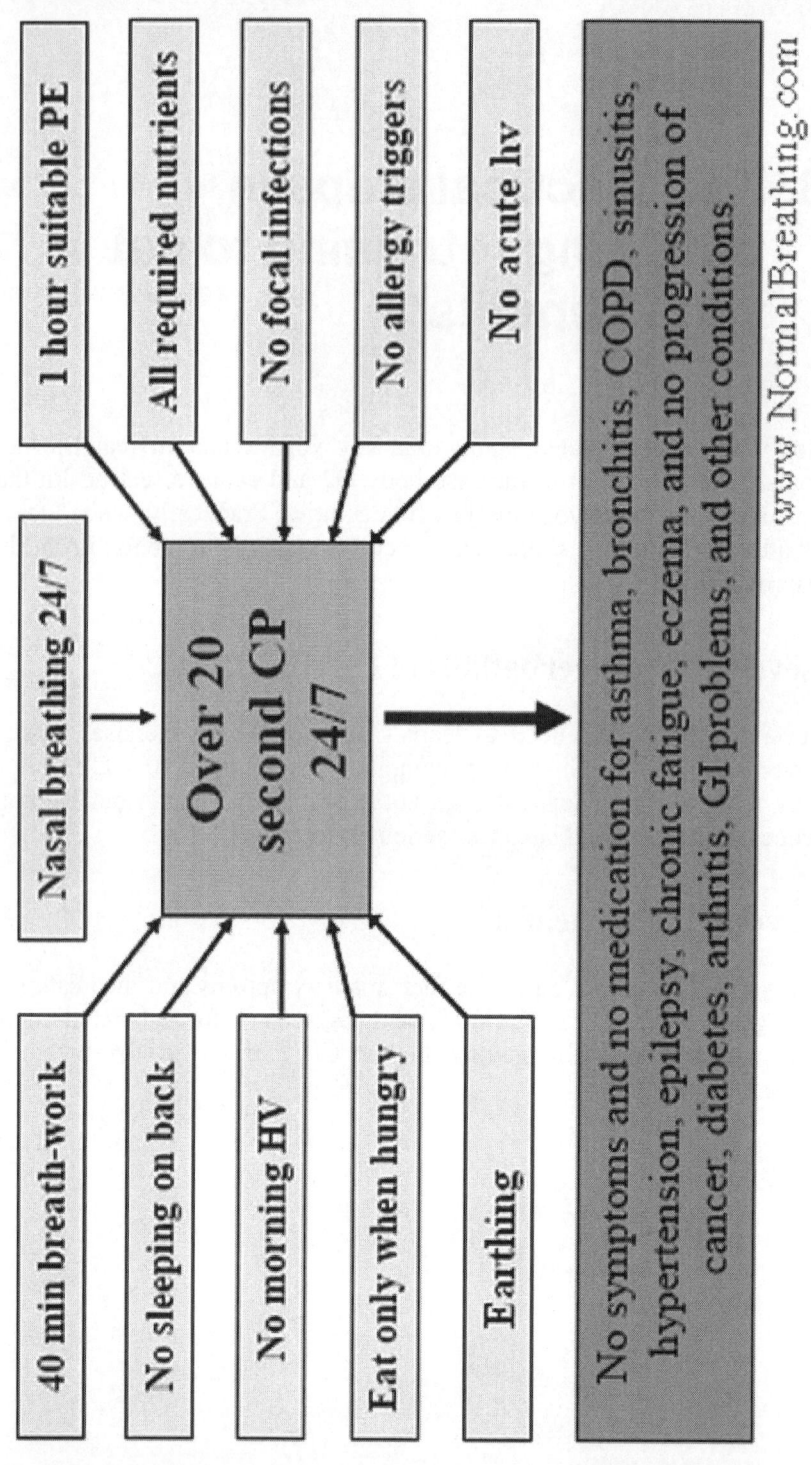

Inputs to Over 20 second CP 24/7

- 1 hour suitable PE
- All required nutrients
- No focal infections
- No allergy triggers
- No acute hv
- Nasal breathing 24/7
- 40 min breath-work
- No sleeping on back
- No morning HV
- Eat only when hungry
- Earthing

Over 20 second CP 24/7 →

No symptoms and no medication for asthma, bronchitis, COPD, sinusitis, hypertension, epilepsy, chronic fatigue, eczema, and no progression of cancer, diabetes, arthritis, GI problems, and other conditions.

www.NormalBreathing.com

Explanations and notes.

Very few people require additional hormonal support (cortisol, thyroxin, etc.) in order to get over 20 second CP. Sometimes, it is necessary to temporarily interrupt some activities that involve hours of hyperventilation. For example, if a person sings or speaks (lectures) every day for 5 or more hours, then these periods of overbreathing may prevent the person from getting over 20 seconds MCP. Such people often require a temporary break to focus on their health. Later, when they get over 20 or more second CP 24/7, they can resume such favorite or desired activities with greatly improved quality. Let us consider these factors in more detail.

A 40 min breath-work program can include 2 breathing sessions each 20 min long, or 3 sessions about 13-14 min long, or 4 sessions at 10 min each.

Among other most fundamental steps are **Prevention of breathing through the mouth** and **Prevention of sleeping on one's back**. There are 2 manuals that can be used, if relevant: Manual "How to prevent sleeping on one's back" and Manual "How to maintain nasal breathing 24/7". They are both provided in the next sections of this book.

No morning HV means no morning hyperventilation (i.e., the CP drop throughout the night should be no more than 5 seconds, preferably less than 3 s). Hence, you have to solve all problems that cause your overnight CP drop.

1 hour suitable PE means 1 hour of total Physical Exercise every day with strictly nasal breathing (in and out) all the time. Usually, less than 20 seconds current CP means feeling tired and inability to do running, jogging, or any other rigorous exercise with strictly nasal breathing for most people. However, walking is possible. Moreover, with further CP increase, students feel empowered and surprised by energy and skills previously hidden in their sick bodies. The initial requirement for physical exercise is to have at least 1 hour every day in total.

All required nutrients are partially considered in the big book "Normal breathing: the key to vital health" and in the manual "Your guide to nutrients that improve breathing and body oxygenation" (to be available soon). The most common deficiencies include fish oil, calcium, magnesium, zinc, and protein. Some other nutritional deficiencies can also slow down or even halt breathing training. Mild cortisol deficiency can also be corrected using a special nutritional support described in the manual.

"**Eat only when hungry**" is the central common sense rule developed by Dr. Buteyko in relation to meals. It also means that you should stop eating at first signs of satiety.

Note for overweight and obese people. *If you are overweight and crave for or are eager to eat fats (except fish oil) or starchy foods (bread, rice, potatoes, etc), you are hyperventilating. Instead of eating, do another breathing session to normalize your blood glucose level and reduce your hunger pangs. If you eat any calorie-rich foods, your CP will get further down. Your progress will be linked to your weight loss. Breathing exercises naturally increase blood glucose levels so that you can feel no hunger for calorie-rich foods. You can surely enjoy all other foods, like vegetables, greens, some fruits, lean meat, fat-free dairy, beans and lentils, etc., if they are a part of your usual diet.*

No focal infections require your analysis or certain health conditions which can not be solved using breathing training only. For example, if you have large intestinal parasites, depending on the toxic load, your current CP will be restricted by 25-35 seconds. There are 4 focal infections:

1. Large intestinal parasites (roundworms, flatworms, hookworms, liver flukes, etc.)
2. Dental cavities (caries or pathogenic anaerobes in teeth)
3. Dead tonsils (degenerated tonsils that do not have blood supply and harbor pathogenic bacteria)
4. Feet mycosis (or athlete's foot).

Sometimes, presence of root canals or mercury amalgams can become the main issue that requires radical solutions for higher CP. More details about focal infections can be found below.

No allergy triggers involves avoidance of any triggers of your allergic responses. These triggers may include:

- air-born dust mites, cat and dog proteins, mold, pollen, paper ink, chemicals, pollutants, and fumes;
- digested gluten products, dairy products, peanuts, tomatoes, and many other foods and substances;
- tap water or other consumed liquids with chemical triggers present;

- substances and objects that can produce an allergic response due to skin contact (synthetic clothes, detergents, paints, metals, plastics, etc.);
- electromagnetic and other penetrating radiation.

Regular allergic inflammatory response exhausts cortisol reserves and suppresses the immune system making breathing normalization very difficult or even impossible.

Earthing or electrical grounding is an additional positive factor that made traditional yoga very powerful against diseases since it increases body O2. It provides free electrons for the human body. Many people found this technique beneficial since it helps to slow down breathing and increase one's CP (often by 2 or more seconds). Earthing counteracts inflammation, psychological stress, muscle pain, back pain and other problems. How does it work?

The human body has a tendency to accumulate positive electrical charge (up to many 100 or 1,000s Volts), while Earth has a slightly negative electrical charge (or excess of electrons). Since many antioxidants, like vitamin C, are able to dis-activate free radicals by donating to them electrons, Earthing can produce a similar effect as antioxidants.

The technique can be used for some part of the day or during sleep. Yoga should be practiced barefoot on soil. This is an important requirement to make yoga more effective. Sleep grounding is another suggested method especially for those people who have low morning CP. One can make simple DIY devices for using Earthing during sleep. The same or similar devices can be applied during daytime.

As a simplest solution, you can get electrically connected (or grounded) with Earth using copper cables that can be found in electrical stores. One end of this cable can be attached to plumbing tubes and another to a small piece of copper that you can keep in your socks (on your feet) during sleep. You can find more ideas, suggestions, ad links on this web page: Earthing (http://www.normalbreathing.com/e/earthing.php) and How to Ground Yourself (http://www.normalbreathing.com/e/how-to-ground-yourself.php).

Other factors

There are many other life-style factors that can significantly influence one's CP progress. For example, prolonged sun-bathing (up to 30 min or more) causes most humans to hyperventilate lowering their CP. Taking a cold shower, on the other hand, is great for helping to achieve normalization of your breathing. There are, however, several necessary safety rules to follow. The most important one is to have over 20 second for the current CP. (More details can be found on the web page "Who and when can safely take cold shower" - http://www.normalbreathing.com/l-cold-shower.php).

Level 3. Normal health

Normal health starts when one gets up to 50 or more for their morning CP. Soviet and Russian Buteyko doctors discovered that, for most people, the most difficult challenge in breathing retraining is to get more than 40 seconds for the morning CP. Most people progress steadily up to about 32-36 s morning CP while using breathing exercises, physical activity and lifestyle changes. However, they cannot advance beyond these numbers.

Conclusions

According to my experience with hundreds of my students, over 90% of people are able to achieve great health and get amazing health benefits if they are able to improve their CP. The same relates to those people who apply yoga correctly. If you already practice yoga, you can surely realize that you can greatly increase your personal yoga benefits, if you start reducing your breathing and holding your breath (if breath holding is safe for you) when practicing asanas and at other times.

However, there are many other methods, tricks, and techniques that are required to get high body O2. Ancient yogi knew how to get there and they tried their best to pass their knowledge to next generations. But they could not anticipate those circumstances and changes that we have on Earth now.

Therefore, if you incorporate correct yoga lifestyle and correct yoga breathing exercises in your practice, you can become a real yoga master.

Printed in Great Britain
by Amazon.co.uk, Ltd.,
Marston Gate.